HERPETIC INFECTIONS OF MAN

HERPETIC
INFECTIONS OF MAN

BY MIRO JURETIĆ, M. D.

with contributions by
VLASTA LINIĆ-VLAHOVIĆ, MILJEN GAZDIK, M.D., AND
VINKO RIBARIĆ, M.D.

UNIVERSITY PRESS OF NEW ENGLAND
HANOVER, NEW HAMPSHIRE

Prepared under the special Foreign Currency Program of the National Library
of Medicine, National Institutes of Health, Public Health Service, U.S. De-
partment of Health, Education, and Welfare, and published for the National
Library of Medicine pursuant to an agreement with the National Science
Foundation, Washington, D.C., by the Nolit Publishing House, Terazije 27/II,
Belgrade, Yugoslavia, 1980. Printed in Yugoslavia.

CONTENTS

AUTHOR:

MIRO JURETIĆ

Ph.D., Pediatrician, Professor of Pediatrics, Medical Faculty, University of Rijeka, Yugoslavia; Chairman, Kantrida Pediatric Clinic, Children's Hospital, Rijeka

CONTRIBUTORS:

VLASTA LINIĆ-VLAHOVIĆ

Ph.D., Associate Professor of Immunology, Department of Physiology, Medical Faculty, University of Rijeka

VINKO RIBARIĆ

M.D., Ph.D., Associate Professor of Ophthalmology, Clinic of Ophthalmology, Sobol General Hospital, Rijeka

MILJEN GAZDIK

M.D., M.Sc., Physician, Kantrida Pediatric Clinic, Children's Hospital, Rijeka

ABBREVIATIONS

ALS: antilymphocyte serum
AMS: antimacrophage serum
ara-A: adenin arabinoside
ara-C: cytosine arabinoside (cytarabine)
CNS: central nervous system
DIC: disseminated intravascular coagulation
DMSO: dimethylsulfoxide
DNA: deoxyribonucleic acid
EBV: Epstein-Barr virus
EEM: erythema exudativum multiforme
EMCV: encephalomyocarditis virus
FPA: p-fluorophenylalanine
HSV: herpes simplex virus
HVH: herpesvirus hominis
IDU:. 5-iodo-2-deoxyuridine
IgM: immunoglobulin M
LT: lymphotoxin
MIF: migration inhibitory factor
Poly-IC: polyinosinic-cydilic acid
RNA: ribonucleic acid
V.A.: (virus) antibody

PREFACE

The increasing importance of the herpes virus group in human and animal pathology has led to the appearance of numerous publications on this theme. I have tried to present some selected chapters concerning the clinical importance of herpetic infection. Some of the topics are selected arbitrarily according to my own field of interest. Although I have been chiefly concerned with primary herpetic infection, which is of great importance in pediatrics, I felt bound to write something about recurrent herpes too, because they are causally connected. I have not dealt with the biology of the herpes virus, because this a chapter which should be written by an author specialized in this field. I have tried to avoid reiterating generally known facts concerning herpes virus infection which can be found in practically all textbooks. Predominantly I have referred to the recently published literature, although I considered it necessary to add certain historic data at the beginning of some chapters. I have tried to emphasize the latest trends in the development of knowledge concerning the herpes virus disease, with some critical evaluation of the results.

I would like to take this opportunity to thank all my collaborators, particularly V. Linić-Vlahović, who greatly helped me with her work and advice. I also wish to express my appreciation to Prof. Mc Nair Scott from Philadelphia for his continuing interest and encouragement. I am especially grateful to my secretary Nevenka Žic for her unstinting work for this publication.

M. Albahari 2. Rijeka   M. Juretić

L'herpès simplex, maladie toute simple! Qui n'a pas eu au cours de sa vie un petit bouton à la lisière de la muqueuse de lèvres et de la peau transformé rapidement en un petit croute et dont il ne s'est pas soucié? Tel est l'herpès simplex, maladie bien commune, à peine une maladie, pourquoi venir vous en parler?

R. Debré, 1958

HERPETIC INFECTIONS OF MAN

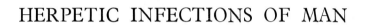

Chapter 1

INTRODUCTION

The Roman physician Herodotus was the first to describe herpetic lesions around the mouth in association with fever, and the term "herpes" had been used in early Greek medicine (ἕρπης to creep) to denote the spreading of different kinds of skin lesions. In the book *De morbis venereis*, the French physician Jean Astruc (1736) first described genital herpetic lesions (cit. by Hutfield 1968). During the 19th century, when modern clinical medicine was born, the word "herpes" was used for all vesicular cutaneous and mucous lesions. By the end of the century the German physician Unna (1883) had made use of a histologic approach to differentiate between pox virus infections and herpesvirus infections. Grüter (1920) and Löwenstein (1919) succeeded in transferring the infection to the rabbit cornea and in identifying herpesvirus hominis as the causative agent of labial herpes and herpetic keratoconjunctivitis. Intranuclear inclusions had been observed in a number of virus infections but Lipschütz (1921) equated the inclusions in herpes simplex with those seen in herpes zoster. In 1934, Cowdry distinguished two types of intranuclear inclusion (A and B) and demonstrated that type A inclusions were pathognomonic for herpesvirus infection. Levaditi (1926) included herpesvirus among the ectodermoses neurotropes and differentiated between herpes simplex and herpes zoster. Andrews and Carmichael (1930) were the first to describe herpetic antibodies in the blood of adults. The American pathologist Hass (1935) correctly described generalized herpes infection in the premature newborn. In 1933, Dawson published his results dealing with encephalitis associated with intranuclear A inclusions. Smith *et al.* (1941) succeeded in isolating herpesvirus from the human brain. Herpes infection was recognized as a common contagious disease as the result of epidemiologic research carried out by Dodd *et al.* (1938) in the United States, by Burnet and Williams (1939) in Australia and by Scott *et al.* (1941) and Black (1942) in the United States. Lipschütz (1921, 1923) was the first to attempt to prove that labial and genital herpes were caused by biologically similar but not identical viruses. His hypothesis was not recognized for some time. During the last 15 years, research by German, Russian and especially American scientists has established the existence of two types of herpesvirus with different biologic properties and antigenic characteristics (Wildy 1973).

Herpesvirus hominis (HVH) type 1 usually prefers an oral localization, whereas HVH type 2 is located predominantly on the genital organs. Infections caused by HVH type 1 are usually located above the waist, whereas clinical manifestations caused by type 2 are usually below the waist. The major epidemiologic difference is the mode of entry for the infection, which is mainly oral for HVH type 1 and usually genital for HVH type 2 (transmitted venereally or from mother to newborn). Herpesvirus type 1 produces smaller colonies when inoculated on chorioallantoic membrane of chick embryo; it is also less neurotropic in inoculation experiments on mice (Shubladze and Chzhu-Shan 1959; Schneweis 1962; Nahmias and Dowdle 1968; Amstey and Balduzzi 1970).

During the last few decades many new viruses from the herpes group (more than 50) have been discovered. More than 30 animal species have been found to be hosts for these viruses. Besides herpes simplex virus (herpesvirus hominis), the greatest importance in human pathology can be attributed to herpesvirus varicellae, cytomegalus virus, Epstein-Barr virus and, to a certain degree, herpesvirus simiae.

Viruses of the herpes types are large viruses with complex structure. Herpesvirus hominis consists of three structural elements. The viral nucleus contains a double helix of deoxyribonucleic acid (DNA). The DNA is located in icosahedral capsids having 162 capsomeres. Infective virions acquire their envelope, containing lipids and glycoproteins, by budding from the nuclear membrane of the cell. The diameter of a complete virion is from 180 to 250 millimicrons (Wildy et al. 1960, Epstein 1967, Chitwood 1970).

Studies made with the electron microscope have helped to elucidate the complex processes that take place after infection with herpesvirus. The interaction between the virion and the cell results in cell degeneration or formation of polycarions ("cythopathogenic effect"). The histologic characteristic of HVH infection is the creation of Lipschütz-Cowdry-type inclusions in infected cells.

Stained inclusions appear as an eosinophilic mass in the nucleus of the cell surrounded by a bright halo. Nuclear chromatin is pushed up against the nuclear membrane at the periphery of the nucleus. The eosinophilic aggregates are probably associated with the process of viral replication. They can be found in the cell a few hours after infection. The formation of polykariocytes is a common consequence of infection with viruses of several different groups. However, polykariocyte formation is especially prominent in infection by the herpesvirus group (Collory 1934; Darlington and Granoff 1973).

The interaction between the virion and the cell can usually be divided into several stages. The first event in this process is the adsorption of the virion at the cell membrane. Its penetration into the cell is associated with the action of specific enzymes and with certain biophysical conditions. In the cell cytoplasm the virion loses its envelope and the liberated nucleocapsid is transported to the nucleus. In the nucleus, viral DNA becomes transcribed. The RNA transcripts are transported to the cytoplasm where they direct the synthesis of virus-specific structural and nonstructural proteins. The structural proteins of the virus migrate back to the nucleus and aggregate with DNA to form the capsid. Capsids become enveloped at the inner nuclear membrane.

During the process of envelopment some membrane-bound viral proteins associate themselves with the viral envelope. It seems that infectivity of the virion is connected with the existence of the viral envelope. Infective virions migrate to the surface of the cell from where they may be released into the medium. The release of viruses into the medium provides a hallmark for the classification of herpes viruses. Herpesvirus hominis belongs to group A, viruses that are, as a rule, released into the medium. The viruses varicella-zoster and cytomegalovirus are examples of group B, which are released into the medium only rarely or not at all (Watson 1973; Nahmias and Roizman 1973; Švara et. al. 1974).

The production of virus by infected human cells is impressive. It is estimated that 80 000 to 120 000 copies of viral DNA are made per cell. The biosynthesis of infectious virion progeny lasts 3 to 5 hours from the moment of infection; this period is called the noninfective phase. Subsequently, in the infective exponential phase there is a rise then a slow drop in infectivity. This type of infection is called *productive infection*. It is best demonstrated in cell culture experiments. Productive infection results in the production of viral progeny capable of infecting other cells, and in cell death. It is responsible for all forms of clinical herpetic diseases, from subclinical to fatal (Nahmias and Roizman 1973).

The other possibility is *nonproductive infection* of the cell, resulting in the perpetuation of the viral genome and survival of the cell. Nonproductive infection is responsible for the phenomenon of recurrent infection. For the majority of patients the origin of the virus that causes recurrent infection is not always clear. Several possibilities for the origin of nonproductive infection have been suggested: exogenous infection, endogenous infection from some other part of the body, chronic continuous multiplication of viruses at the place of infection, persistence of the viral genome at reduced levels in the nonproductive form at or near the place of infection. It has been hypothesized that the places of persistence of HVH are epithelial cells or sensory ganglion cells of the nerve endings, where recurrent lesions occur (Baringer 1975). A more recent hypothesis also suggests the persistence of HVH in the exocrine glands of the majority of adults (lacrimal gland, prostate, and vesicula seminalis; Centifanto *et al.* 1972).

Herpesvirus hominis is an ectodermal parasite with man as its only host. Predilected places of infection are the skin, mucous membranes, eyes and brain. On certain occasions the virus develops pantropism, which mostly affects visceral organs. This occurs chiefly in instances of decreased resistance in the young organism (prematurity, kwashiorkor, immunologic defects, and the like). A sensitive person is usually infected during childhood with HVH type 1 on the occasion of the first exposure to the fairly widespread virus. This is *primary* or *initial infection,* which is usually subclinical.

It has been established that 10 to 20 percent of all infected children show clinical sings of primary infection, mainly evident as acute gingivostomatitis herpetica (Juretić, 1966). After the initial infection antibodies against HVH type 1 are developed in the serum and more or less persist throughout life. Primary infection with HVH type 2 occurs most often in adults following puberty, usually by venereal contact, after which specific antibodies develop in the organism. After the primary infection, both herpesviruses persist in the host organism in latent form. Different factors may disturb the equilibrium, so that older persons, in particular, may experience exacerbation of herpetic infection, which is called *secondary recurrent infection.*

Chapter 2

EPIDEMIOLOGY*

I. Reservoir of virus and transmission of infection

The reservoir of herpesvirus hominis (HVH) is man himself. The continued presence of herpesvirus in the population is a well-established fact. Most infections by this virus appear to be subclinical; it has been estimated that 80 to 90 percent of these infections fall into this category (Scott 1954, 1957; Juretić 1966).

Sources of herpetic infection are: (1) other patients, mainly children, with primary disease; (2) adults with recurrent exacerbation; (3) children as healthy carriers — about 20 percent, according to Buddingh *et al.* (1953); (4) adults as healthy carriers — about 2 percent, again according to Buddingh *et al.* (1953).

A 6-year study of the epidemiology of virus infection in a children's home, made by Cesario *et al.* (1969), revealed that 32.1 percent of the children shed HVH at least once. The majority of the isolates were not associated with primary infections. Episodes of non-primary virus shedding came at varying intervals and lasted about 5 months.

In 1960, Burnet concluded that "in the intervals between eruptions, the virus must remain latent in the epidermal cells of the affected areas of the skin..." The cells concerned must be deeper layers of the skin epithelium which continually multiply to maintain the epidermal structure.

It has subsequently been suggested that it is chronic infection of lacrimal and salivary glands with HVH which provides the source of virus for recurrent herpetic lesions, rather than activation of latent virus in nerve cells or epithelial cells at the site of recurrent lesions (Kaufman *et al.* 1967). This contention is supported by the demonstration of HVH in lacrimal glands of infected rabbits, and the consistent finding in animals and man of HVH in tears and saliva in the absence of herpetic lesions (Kaufman *et al.* 1968;

---

* This chapter is concerned with the epidemiology of HVH type 1 only. The epidemiology of HVH type 2 is described in chapter 4.

Lindgren *et. al.* 1968). Lindgren and associates found that 5 percent of 418 adults excreted HVH after experimental infection of the nose.

However, data obtained in a study by Douglas and Couch show that the parotid glands were not infected with HVH; other salivary and mucous glands may have been the source of herpesvirus (1970). Previously reported rates of HVH isolation were determined by cross-sectional epidemiologic surveys based on single specimens and are not entirely reliable. It is interesting that in a prospective study by Douglas and Couch, 8 out of 10 normal adults had HVH in oral secretions at least once when cultured twice weekly over 5 months.

Recently, latently infected sensory ganglia have been thought to be the source of virus for various clinical manifestations of recurrent herpetic disease in man. Stevens and Cook showed that HVH can induce a latent infection in the spinal ganglia of mice (1971). Nesburn, Cook and Stevens (1972) have found that latent HVH is present in trigeminal ganglions of rabbits with recurrent ocular infection. This finding further supports the concept that in man sensory ganglia are the reservoir of HVH in the period between exacerbations of overt disease. Baringer and Swoveland (1973) have convincingly demonstrated that the repressed HVH genome can be recovered from human trigeminal ganglions infected with herpes simplex virus. Later, the virus was found in sacral and lumbar sensory ganglions (Baringer 1974, 1975; Bastian *et al.* 1972; Finelli and McDonald 1975).

Baringer (1975) concluded "that this virus may have the capability to reside in a wide variety of sensory ganglion cells of which the trigeminal and third and fourth sacral are only the most frequent", because oral and genital mucosas are common sites for primary and recurrent herpes lesions."

The appearance of herpetic lesions in the skin areas supplied by the sectioned portion of the trigeminal nerve root (Cushing, quoted by Constantine *et al.* 1969; Carton and Kilbourne 1952) suggests the possibility of another source of latent virus.

Transmission of HVH type 1 infections appears to occur primarily by direct contact, most likely by way of the saliva or oral secretions (Buddingh *et al.* 1953) Probably close personal contact as in kissing or wrestling for example is needed (Selling and Kibrick 1964; Porter and Baughman 1965). Herpesvirus, like Epstein-Barr virus, has been named the "virus of love." This mode of propagation may account for the outbreaks of gingivostomatitis herpetica reported from families and other closed populations (Burnet and Wiliams 1939; Scott *et al.* 1950; Chilton 1944; Anderson and Hamilton 1949; Juretić 1960; Hale *et al.* 1963; Piringer 1958).

Possible ways of virus transmission by air (droplets) or via infected skin scrames are not well documented. The distribution of infections all the year round, a pronounced correlation between the disease and socio-economic conditions, a great number of isolated cases, and sizeable epidemics, all speak very convincingly for transmission by direct contact. Early childhood abounds in numerous close contacts either through kissing or through chewing utensils. Quite certainly, all kinds of injuries may also favor infection by herpesvirus. Thus "herpes traumaticus" may result from injuries occurring during dentition, and from skin lesions caused by burns or abrasions (*Brit. Med. J.* 1970).

Spreading of the virus by saliva is confirmed by the cases of herpetic paronychia in medical and dental personnel who handle infected oral cavity patients or contaminated tracheal catheters (Stern *et al.* 1959; Rosato *et al.* 1970). Medical and nursing personnel particularly risk primary HVH infection, because less than 50 percent of them have HVH antibodies in their sera (Nahmias and Roizman 1973). The spread of HVH by sexual intercourse is described in Chapter 4.

The percentage of *contacts* reported varies widely. Most of the reports are based on a small number of observed cases. Black, observing 80 patients, found contact with herpetic infection in only 10 percent. Spence and collaborators proved the source of infection in 17 out 64 patients, or in 27 percent. Scott, admittedly in the lowest number of patients (21) reported 10 contacts, i.e. 50 percent (1957). In our survey (Juretić 1970) of 581 patients with primary herpetic disease *the source of infection was found in 158 (27.2 percent)*. In one half of all contacts recurrent herpetic infection of adults proved to be the source of infection. In the other half the source of infection was other children with primary herpetic disease. There is no doubt that a certain number of children were infected by healthy carriers. There are obvious difficulties in establishing the source of infection for a child who already has a certain social life and may have had a great number of passing contacts. *The more carefully one looks for the cause of infection, the more frequently is the cause found to be an adult with exacerbation of herpetic infection.* This opinion is substantiated by frequent reports in the literature of eczema herpeticum and neonatal herpes where the history of contacts was looked into thoroughly and the primary source was far more frequently found to be an adult. Despite the presence of high levels of neutralising antibody, herpes labialis often recurs in adults. Antibody and virus coexist and this results in the formation of infectious virus-antibody (V.A.) complexes. The existence of such complexes in human recurrent herpetic lesions has been demonstrated. Patients with active lesions shed high concentrations of virus and that natural infection may be transmitteed by an infectious V. A. complex (Daniels *et al.*, 1975).

II Age and sex distribution; seasonal and long-term trend

A correlation exists between the level of neutralizing and complement fixing antibodies in the population and susceptibility to infection with herpesvirus (HVH). The period of greatest susceptibility comes after the cessation of maternal postpartal protection of the child. During the first 6 months of life, transplacental HVH antibodies can be detected in the sera of newborns whose mothers had HVH antibodies. Offspring of mothers without antibodies (both types) are exceptionally susceptible from birth and represent the rare group exhibiting the very serious form of herpetic infection, neonatal herpes. From 6 months to 2 years only a few children have this protection. A sharp rise of antibodies against type 1 herpesvirus takes place between 1 and 4 years. This is the period in which most initial infection with HVH type 1 occurs (Fig. 1), with the mouth as the most common site of herpetic involvement.

Other forms of clinically evident primary infection such as eczema herpeticum, herpes cutis, herpes digitorum, and genital herpes are less frequent in this age period.

Gingivostomatitis herpetica has its peak incidence in the second year of life. In case material from Split (Yugoslavia) the incidence of the disease fell off steeply after the third year so that by school age only a few isolated cases were recorded. The graph in Fig. 1 shows this age distribution.

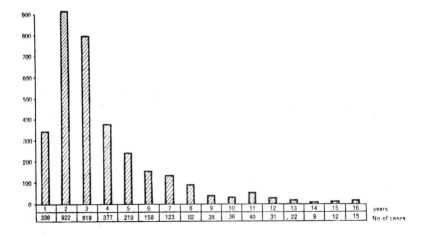

Fig. 1. Age distribution of 3278 cases of primary herpetic infection in the city of Split 1952—1962 (Juretić 1966).

There was very similar age distribution in 92 cases of fatal postneonatal herpetic dissemination in South Africa (Kipps *et al.* 1967).

The age distribution of herpes ophthalmicus is somewhat different from that of the other forms of herpetic infection, the highest incidence being in the 41 to 60 year age group (Gold *et al.* 1965).

The incidence of genital herpes and of herpes encephalitis is described in Chapters 4 and 9.

Sex distribution is almost the same in all forms of herpetic infection.

The incidence of primary herpetic infection does not exhibit *seasonal variations* (Fig. 2). Gingivostomatitis herpetica appears to be one of the most evenly distributed diseases with the regard to season. HVH infections of the skin occur more commonly in the warmer months, whereas HVH infections of the eye and herpes labialis seem to be more frequent in winter (Nahmias 1972). There was no clear seasonal variation in the incidence of fatal herpes infection in South Africa (Becker 1966).

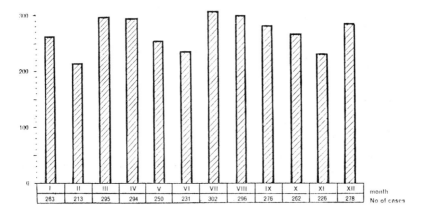

Fig.2. Seasonal distribution of 3186 cases of primary herpetic infection in the city of Split (1952—1962). (Juretić 1966).

Herpetic infection does not show any special *long term fluctuations* either. This can be seen from Fig. 3, which gives the incidence of gingivostomatitis herpetica in a 10-year period. Minor fluctations are attributable to the accumulation of cases in families and institutions and do not indicate epidemics.

No seasonal or long term fluctuation in the prevalence of HVH was observed during a 2-year respiratory virus survey in four villages in West Bengal (Kloene *et al.* 1970). The virus isolations were more or less evenly distributed over the study period.

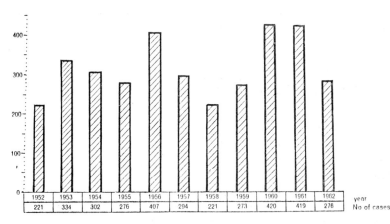

	1952	1953	1954	1955	1956	1957	1958	1959	1960	1961	1962	year
	221	334	302	276	407	294	221	273	420	419	276	No of cases

Fig. 3. Long term trend of the incidence of primary herpetic infection in the city of Split (1952—1962). Analysis of 3443 cases. (Juretić 1966).

III Incubation

Serial investigations of the incubation perid of herpetic infections are rather few. In 1957 Scott published 33 cases in which the incubation period varied from 3 to 9 days. In the literature there are many individual observations regarding the incubation period, all of which fall within the above range.

From Fig. 4 it may be seen that the incubation period varied from 2 to 12 days with an arithmetic mean of 6.1 days (Juretić 1960). The clinical impression is that shorter incubation periods, from 4 to 6 days are more frequent. Hale *et al.* (1963) has reported a small epidemic of herpetic gingivostomatitis with a similar incubation period of 6 to 8 days. The wider span of 2 to 20 days cited by Nahmias and Roizman (1973) is not probable.

The incubation period of HVH encephalitis is more difficult to define but it appears to be longer (Nahmias and Roizman 1973).

The incubation period of genital herpes and particularly of neonatal herpes is cited in Chapters 4 and 5.

IV Incidence of manifest herpetic infection; epidemics of herpetic disease

The study of the incidence of manifest herpetic infection presents considerable difficulties. The incidence of primary herpetic disease, which could be called the attack rate, depends to a certain extent on the sample of subjects examined and, naturally, on the thoroughness, duration and continuity of the observation.

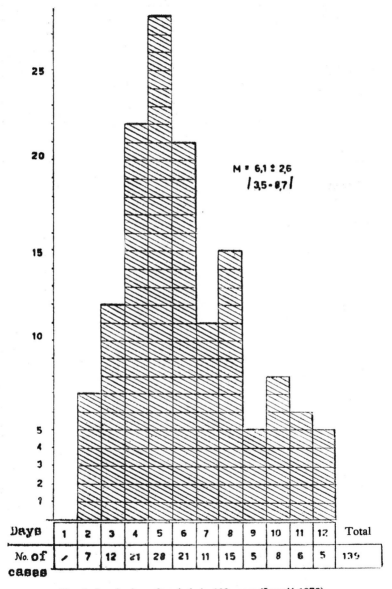

Fig. 4. Incubation of periods in 139 cases (Juretić 1970).

Blank and Rake (1954) state that only 1 of 500 persons suffered from manifest infection, i.e. 0.2 percent. Scott (1957) reports that 38 out of 5016 children, or 0.8 percent had herpetic disease. A cohort study carried out by Spence et al. (1954) in England showed that 65 out of 950 children (6.8 percent) followed up during a period of 5 years were manifestly ill.

In a survey lasting more than 5 years of 14 539 children from Split, Yugoslavia, the attack rate of clinically evident herpetic infection was found to be 13.2 percent. The frequency was conspicuously lower in various age groups observed for a shorter period of time. At least 10—15 percent of all children got the disease by the age of 9 (Juretić 1966). A part of the study is presented in Table 1.

Table 1. *Incidence of manifest herpetic infection in Split*

Year of birth	Number of children examined	Number of children with disease	Duration of observation (years)	Percentage of children with disease
1955	936	123	9	13.4
1956	935	131	8	14.8
1957	870	119	7	13.8
1958	1450	136	6	9.4
Total	4191	509		12.1

The *attack rate* is quite different in cases with high agglomeration in families with many children, in hospitals, nurseries and orphanages.

In 1939, in the addendum to their paper, Burnet and Williams, who contributed greatly to the modern epidemiology of herpetic infection, set forth an interesting example of a *family epidemic* observed by a general practitioner (A.P. Derham). The mother and the housemaid had secondary labial herpes and infected two children; 5 days later the third child fell ill. In 1941 Scott et al. described three separate one-family epidemics. In 1944 Chilton published a herpetic epidemic in a Negro family of eight members.

In Yugoslavia 12 family epidemics have been reported (Juretić 1966). The attack rate was 100 percent i.e. all children (3 or 4) in these families showed manifest disease (Fig. 5). However, further observations with serologic data and more abundant material are needed (Juretić 1960, Juretić and Petković, 1960).

Recently reported small family epidemics in Italy (Copaitich et al. 1972) have not helped to determine what is the exact attack rate in families.

Hospital epidemics of herpetic diseases are more significant. The risk is especially high in concentrations of very suspectible infants with eczema. Ward epidemics of eczema herpeticum are

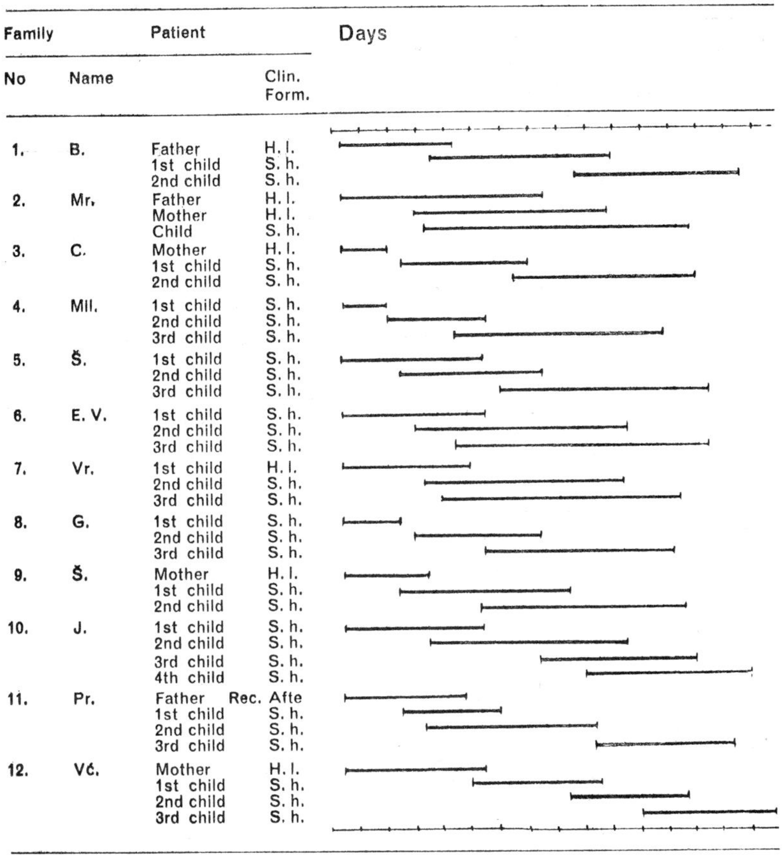

Family		Patient		Days
No	Name		Clin. Form.	
1.	B.	Father	H. l.	
		1st child	S. h.	
		2nd child	S. h.	
2.	Mr.	Father	H. l.	
		Mother	H. l.	
		Child	S. h.	
3.	C.	Mother	H. l.	
		1st child	S. h.	
		2nd child	S. h.	
4.	Mll.	1st child	S. h.	
		2nd child	S. h.	
		3rd child	S. h.	
5.	Š.	1st child	S. h.	
		2nd child	S. h.	
		3rd child	S. h.	
6.	E. V.	1st child	S. h.	
		2nd child	S. h.	
		3rd child	S. h.	
7.	Vr.	1st child	H. l.	
		2nd child	S. h.	
		3rd child	S. h.	
8.	G.	1st child	S. h.	
		2nd child	S. h.	
		3rd child	S. h.	
9.	Š.	Mother	H. l.	
		1st child	S. h.	
		2nd child	S. h.	
10.	J.	1st child	S. h.	
		2nd child	S. h.	
		3rd child	S. h.	
		4th child	S. h.	
11.	Pr.	Father	Rec. Afte	
		1st child	S. h.	
		2nd child	S. h.	
		3rd child	S. h.	
12.	Vć.	Mother	H. l.	
		1st child	S. h.	
		2nd child	S. h.	
		3rd child	S. h.	

Fig. 5. Family epidemics of herpetic infections. S. h. Stomatitis herpetica. H. 1. herpes labialis. |—| Duration of illness. (Juretić 1966).

described in Chapter 8. A large contact epidemic in a Yugoslav children's hospital has been reported (Juretić and Brož 1960). The attack rate among 37 children exposed to this epidemic was found to be 57 percent (Fig. 6). A hospital epidemic has also been reported from Venezuela, with 35 diseased children (Piringer 1958).

Anderson and Hamilton (1949) describe an epidemic among 43 exposed sero-negative infants with 61 percent sero-conversions and 46 percent manifest illness. The duration of observation was one year (1949).

Hale noted an attack rate of clinically apparent herpes simplex infection in 77 percent of 13 children in an orphanage (1963).

Patient					Days
No	Name	months	Clin. form	Ward	
1.	M. S.	10	S. h.	I	
2.	Z. J.	13	S. h.	I	
3.	K. M.	5	S.h.+K.h.	I	
4.	J. D.	11	S. h.	I	
5.	J. M.	7	S.h.+K.h.	I	
6.	S. N.	13	S. h.	I	
7.	P. I.	9	S. h.	I	
8.	J. Z.	8	S. h.	I	
9.	S. M.	19	S.h.+H.c.	II	
10.	B. S.	9	S. h.	I	
11.	K. I.	6	S. h.	II	
12.	P. S.	10	S. h.	I	
13.	V. N.	15	S. h.	III	
14.	K. R.	13	S. h.	III	
15.	K. M.	7	S. h.	I	
16.	B. H.	7	S. h.	I	
17.	D. B.	8	H. c.	I	

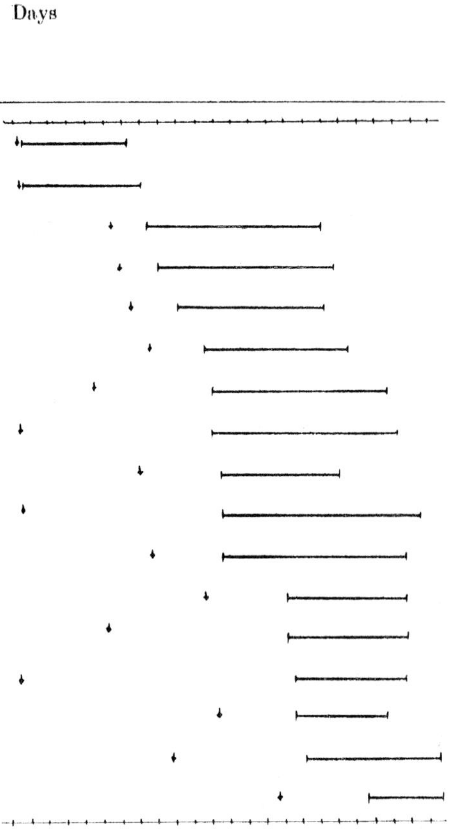

Fig. 6. Hospital epidemic of herpetic infecion. S. h. Stomatitis herpetica. H. c. Herpes cutis. K. h. Keratitis herpeica. |—| Duration of illness. ↓ Admission to Hospital (Juretić 1966).

In three small epidemics in the orphanage of Split the percentage of manifest infections in the majority of the exposed children was very high: 71—83 percent (Juretić 1966). Serologic investigations were not made (Fig. 7). Data published by Cesario *et al.* (1969) give a rather different picture. Their survey revealed that the virus failed to spread to the susceptible inmates of a children's home.

In this population one-half of the children were immune and 32 percent shed virus periodically. Eight of 70 seronegative children (11 percent) converted and only 1 child experienced acute gingivo-stomatitis during 6-year surveillance. Spread of the virus requires

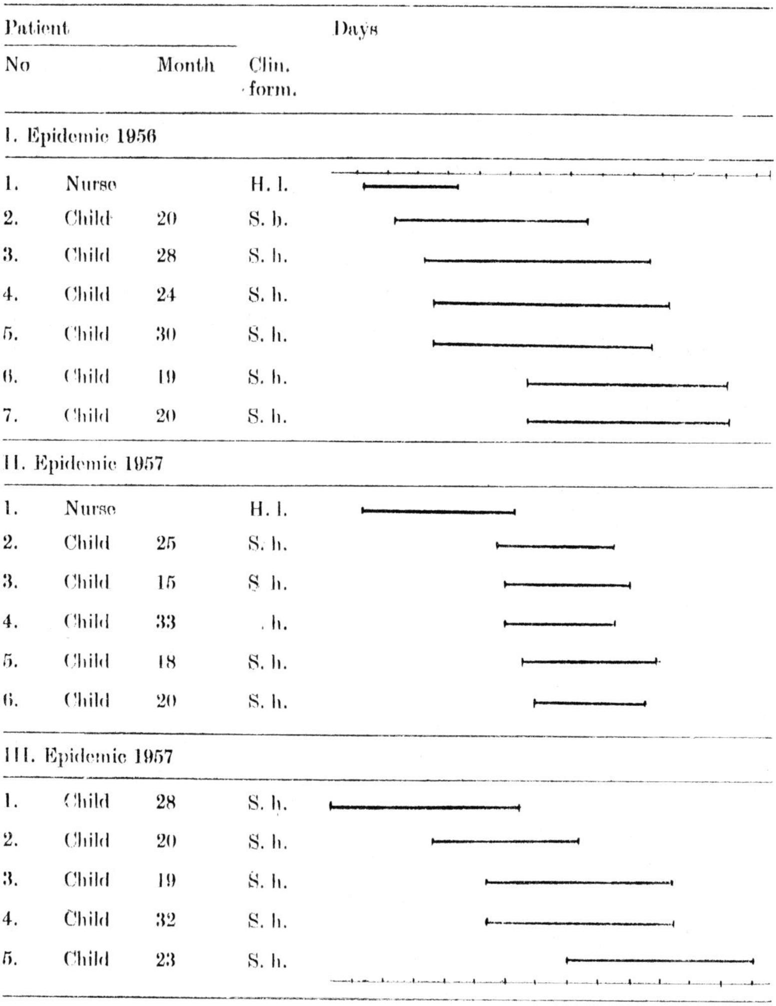

Patient			Days
No	Month	Clin. form.	
I. Epidemic 1956			
1.	Nurse		H. l.
2.	Child	20	S. h.
3.	Child	28	S. h.
4.	Child	24	S. h.
5.	Child	30	S. h.
6.	Child	19	S. h.
7.	Child	20	S. h.
II. Epidemic 1957			
1.	Nurse		H. l.
2.	Child	25	S. h.
3.	Child	15	S h.
4.	Child	33	. h.
5.	Child	18	S. h.
6.	Child	20	S. h.
III. Epidemic 1957			
1.	Child	28	S. h.
2.	Child	20	S. h.
3.	Child	19	S. h.
4.	Child	32	S. h.
5.	Child	23	S. h.

Fig. 7. Institutional epidemics of herpetic infections. S. h. Stomatitis herpetica. H. 1. Herpes labialis. |—| Duration of illness (Juretić 1966).

close and intimate contact. The rate of seroconversion in this study was very similar to the rate of about 10 percent found in university students without antibodies who developed antibodies each year during the period of surveillance (Glezen *et al.* 1975). The correlation between these rates and the attack rate in the general child population (10—15 percent) is evident.

The difference between these results and those of other investigators perhaps arises from the broad age range of the population studied and the fact that Cesario and collaborators made their observations in orphanages in the absence of epidemics. Juretić's study involved epidemics of manifest disease in infants.

In a recent publication Glezen *et al.* (1975) report that infections with HVH type 1 were associated with 11.5 percent of acute respiratory illnesses in students who were admitted to the student infirmary over a 6-year period. Over three-quarters of these infections were found in students with pharyngitis or tonsillitis; many infections were not accompanied by an exudate; 43 percent of the patients had ulcerative lesions on the tonsils or the posterior pharynx but only 11 percent had lesions in the anterior portion of the mouth and lips. A significant antibody rise — primary infection with HVH — was demonstrated in 80 percent of cases.

V Serology of primary herpetic infection; social implications

All systematic investigations suggest a close tie between age and serologic status. They indicate increasing acquisition of HVH antibodies with increasing age, after the disappearance of transplacental antibodies usually within months after birth.

Observations used to be made by neutralization or complement fixation tests using untyped strains of HVH. At that time the population was divided into two groups: herpetic and non herpetic. Now the situation is quite different; there are four distinct population groups according to serum HVH antibodies: (1) without antibodies; (2) with type 1 antibodies; (3) with type 2 antibodies; (4) with antibodies of both types. The dynamics of acquisition of the two antibody types is presented in Fig. 8 of chapter 4.

The distribution of herpesvirus among different groups of the population demonstrates a negative correlation between the rate of acquisition of antibodies and socio-economic status. It seems that the spread of HVH is facilitated by poor hygiene and overcrowding. This was first clearly demonstrated by the study of Burnet and Williams (1939) who obtained 37 percent positive findings among medical students as compared with 93 percent positives among hospital patients. This correlation has been corroborated by several workers (Buddingh, *et al.* 1953, Goetze 1955, Scott 1957). Kibrick and Gooding (1965) report that antibodies of herpesvirus were present in 62 percent of private patients, in 84 percent of ward service patients and in only 30 to 37 percent of college undergraduates and young doctors. The low incidence of antibodies in these young people indicates the possibility of occupational risk of infection from patients and suggests that primary herpetic infection might be encountered more frequently than before in teenagers and young adults (Smith et al. 1967).

Becker (1966) compared the incidence of HVH antibodies in three groups of the population in Cape Town. They found that it was lower in the white population than in the colored population, and the Bantus had the highest incidence.

Porter et al. (1969) in the United States demonstrated the same correlation between age, income and herpesvirus infections. There were very low rates of positive findings among medical students (20 percent) and laboratory personnel (40 percent). A similar rate among students (30 percent) has recently been reported also in the United States (Glezen et al. 1975)

Infection in the upper social classes tends to occur beyond early childhood and in some populations 40—50 percent of young adults do not have antibodies to the virus. This is demonstrated by the study of Wentworth and Alexander (1971) who determined the prevalence of complement-fixing antibodies to HVH from a predominantly middle class urban population of ages 5 to 60 years. Females had a higher prevalence of HVH antibodies at all ages than did males; the sera from pregnant women had a somewhat greater prevalence, but this increase was not sufficient to account for the difference between male and female rates. More recently it was noted that a change in age distribution had occurred in Japan (Yoshino and Taniguchi 1966).

The decrease in the incidence of herpetic antibodies in a population is perhaps best illustrated by the data obtained from two surveys made in England (Holzel et al. 1953, Smith et al. 1967). This apparent decrease in the incidence of herpetic infection might be attributed to improvement of the social environment, better housing conditions and increased awareness of and facilities for simple hygienic requirements among a larger population (Smith et al. 1967).

Chapter 3

IMMUNOLOGY OF HERPESVIRUS INFECTION

V. LINIĆ-VLAHOVIĆ

With recent advances in immunobiology it has become apparent that a host's resistance to virus infections depends on the working of several distinct specific and nonspecific defense mechanisms. Moreover, the accumulated experimental data suggest that immune responses which participate in the defense against viruses may also play a role in the pathogenesis of certain viral diseases.

I Nonspecific mechanisms

One of the most important nonspecific immune responses to viral antigens is the production of interferon. Interferon is a protein, or rather a family of proteins, produced by cells of various types following interaction with viruses and a variety of nonviral substances. As regards the mechanism of its action, the available information suggests that it interferes with the translation steps in viral replication. The process seems to consist of the induction of a second protein, the active antiviral principle, invoked by the interferon released (De Clercq and Merigan 1970).

There is evidence that herpesvirus promotes interferon production in infected cultured cells (Aurelian and Roizman 1965; Fruitstone *et al.* 1964; Lampson *et al.* 1965). However, the virus appears to be only moderately sensitive to the action of interferon. This was indicated by the early in vitro studies (Isaacs 1961; Brown 1966). But in experiments in vivo, interferon failed to prevent the replication of herpes virus in rabbit cornea (Cantell and Tommila 1960).

More recently, interest has focused on the role of interferon inducers in resistance to infection by viruses including herpesvirus. Since the initial observation by Park and Baron (1968) that synthetic double-stranded ribonucleic acids which induce interferon production promote recovery from herpetic keratitis in rabbits, several other workers have reported the successful use of polynucleotides in herpesvirus infection. Reference to these has been made in connection with the therapy of herpes virus infection. In this context it is pertinent that certain polynucleotides enhance the specific immune responses (Brown *et al.* 1971; Johnson *et al.* 1971). However, the basis for this effect is not clear at present.

Another important mechanism of a host's defense against some infections is the uptake of infectious agent by macrophages. Although the role of macrophages as instruments of antibacterial resistance was recognized long ago, information regarding their capacity to interfere with viruses is only now beginning to accumulate. The results obtained using different approaches, experimental animals and viruses, taken all together, indicate that macrophages prevent the spread of some viruses while serving as potential vehicles for the propagation of others (Panijel and Cayeux 1968; Hirsch *et al.* 1969.). Evidence for the potential host's dependence on macrophages for defense against herpesvirus infection is derived from experimental studies in mice. It has been demonstrated that following intraperitoneal inoculation of herpesvirus into adult mice the virus remains largely associated with peritoneal macrophages, and that treatment of mice with anti-macrophage serum (AMS) prior to virus inoculation increases mortality. Further, it has been shown that adult mouse macrophages protect suckling mice from subsequent intraperitoneal infection with herpesvirus (Johnson, 1964 a, b; Zisman *et al.* 1970; Hirsch *et al.* 1970). Thus, at least in this mammalian species, macrophages have been found to function as an efficient primary barrier against the systemic propagation of the virus. Obviously, the importance of further studies along these lines cannot be underestimated in view of the close association of macrophages with specific, cell-mediated immune reactions.

II Specific mechanisms

Convincing evidence has been obtained indicating that specific resistance to a wide variety of infectious diseases is generated by two distinct mechanisms: humoral and cellular. Moreover, it has become clear that full expression of immunity depends on the cooperative interaction between two distinct lymphoid cell lines. One line is thymus cells (T-cells) and is incapable of producing circulating antibodies. The other, derived from bone marrow, is the progenitor of antibody producing cells (B-cells) and requires collaboration with T-cells to perform its function.

Humoral immunity. Primary infection with herpesvirus stimulates the production of specific neutralizing and complement-fixing antibodies. The presence of these antibodies in animal and human sera can be demonstrated by a variety of serologic techniques, as reviewed recently by Plummer (1973).

Data from numerous sero-epidemiologic surveys in man indicate that about 90 percent of adults have specific herpesvirus antibodies in their serum. They also reveal that there is a marked difference in the distribution of HVH antibodies among different population and different age groups. In general, there is an inverse relation between the incidence of these antibodies and socioeconomic status of the population (Burnet and Lush 1939; Becker 1966). With regard to age distribution, a high antibody incidence was found among newborn and young infants and a very low incidence among older infants and children under the age of about 3 years. The incidence then rises with increasing age and reaches a peak by late adulthood (Smith *et al.* 1967; Nahmias *et al.* 1970b; Gerber and Rosenblum 1968). The presence of herpesvirus antibodies at birth and their subsequent disappearance during the early postnatal period indicates the existence of specific passive immunity acquired by virtue of the placental transfer of maternal antibodies to the fetus. This in turn implies that antibodies transferred across the placenta serve to protect the fetus and neonate from infection with herpesvirus.

Antibodies formed in response to infection by herpesvirus comprise a heterogenous population of gamma-globulin molecules, each with distinct physico-chemical and immunochemical properties. Obvious heterogeneity is manifested by the three major classes of immunoglobulins (IgG, IgM and IgA) containing the antiviral antibody activity. More subtle heterogeneity within the antibody population is displayed by substantial diversity in immunochemical properties. Thus, it has been shown that 7S and 19S herpesvirus antibodies produced at different times after infection differ in their neutralizing properties against isologous and against cross reacting herpes virus strains (Hampar *et al.* 1968a, b, 1970, 1971a, b; Stevens *et al.* 1968). More recent studies have demonstrated that 7S and 19S HVH antibodies fractionated from early and late immune rabbit sera can discriminate between different herpesvirus structural proteins (Miyamoto *et al.* 1971; Hampar *et al.* 1971a). Obviously, herpesvirus is not a simple antigen but a complex structure composed of antigenically distinct parts (Olshevsky and Becker 1970; Keller *et al.* 1970; Roizman *et al.* 1970; Martin *et al.* 1972). These parts or epitopes determine the specificity of the antibody response.

Although individual antibodies to herpes virus have a high degree of specificity, some may show cross-reaction with closely related antigens. Thus, a strong cross-reaction occurs between type 1 and type 2 HVH (Nahmias and Dowdle 1968; Rawls *et al.* 1970b). In the last few years considerable interest has been focused on the antibody response to the two types of herpesvirus. Using microneutralization techniques, several investigators have shown that antibodies produced in response to primary infection with either type 1 or type 2 can be readily distinguished, whereas those formed in response to infection with both HVH types have "dual" or "intermediate" properties (Nahmias *et al.* 1969b; Rawls *et al.* 1970b). There appears to be little doubt that the reason for the occurrence of "intermediate" antibodies resides in antigenic similarities between the two HVH serotypes. Indeed, recent serologic studies with experimental anti-HVH sera have provided evidence indicating that type 1 and type 2 HVH share cross-reacting antigens (Bernstein and Stewart 1971, Martin *et al.* 1972).

Circulating antibody has long been regarded as a major defense mechanism against virus infections. However, although this may be true for systemic infections, it is quite clear that humoral antibodies are incapable of preventing intracellular virus persistence and latent infections. Thus, antibodies to herpes virus do not provide protection against herpes recurrences (Burnet and Lush 1939; Allison 1967). Experimental work has shown that inoculation of herpesvirus into normal skin of persons subject to herpesvirus eruptions may provoke a new area of recurrent infection in spite of the presence of high levels of specific circulating antibody in these persons (Lazar 1956; Goldman 1961).

In vitro studies have also indicated that neutralizing antibody in the culture medium does not alter the behavior of the virus already established in the cultured cells (Wheeler 1960).

Local immunity. Local immunity mediated by secretory IgA antibodies is considered to play an important part in resistance to some virus infections. With respect to herpesvirus infection, the data reported by Scalise *et al.* (1972) seem to indicate that the occurrence of recurrent herpes keratitis in man might be due to a temporary deficiency of local antibody production. However, evidence derived from a more detailed study Centifanto *et al.* (1970) indicates that herpes recurrences are not related to the amount

3*

of secretory IgA antibodies. Similar observations have been reported by Douglas and Couch (1970) who failed to demonstrate a correlation between the concentration of salivary IgA and recurrent herpesvirus infection of the mouth. Nevertheless, in the study of Centifanto et al. (1970), topical immunization of rabbit eye with heat-inactivated herpesvirus resulted in the production of secretory IgA antibodies that were capable of neutralizing HVH in vitro and protecting the animal from initial infection. In an extension of their study, Centifanto and Kaufman (1970) obtained evidence suggesting that the effective neutralization of herpesvirus in ocular tissue may depend on the relative concentrations of IgA and IgG antibodies. They found that virus sensitized with IgG antibodies is protected from neutralization by IgA antibody, and that larger amounts of IgA antibody are required to neutralize the sensitized virus. However it still cannot be said with certainty what is the actual protective value of exocrine IgA antibody in primary HVH infection and recurrences.

Cell-mediated immunity. A great deal of evidence indicates that T-cell-mediated immune responses play an essential role in the expression of specific resistance to many virus infections. The host's dependence on these responses for defense against herpesvirus infection is illustrated by a number of clinical and experimental findings. Clinical experience has shown that the virus produces severe, often fatal infection in patients with congenital thymus deficiency syndromes (St. Geme et al. 1965; Cooper et al. 1968; Kretsch et al. 1969; Sutton et al. 1974). Similar observations have been made in patients receiving antilymphocyte serum (ALS) or other immunosuppressive agents (Schwartz 1969; Montgomerie et al. 1969; Russell 1974). Further, it has been reported that individuals with severe protein malnutrition, such as kwashiorkor, are also prone to the development of severe herpesvirus infection (McKenzie et al. 1959; Templeton, 1970). In this condition a defective cell-mediated immune response seems to be involved (Smythe et al. 1971).

These observations on human patients are well supported by experimental studies. Thus, depression of cell-mediated immunity by neonatal thymectomy or ALS administration has been shown to increase the severity of herpesvirus infection in mice (Mori 1967; Zisman et al. 1970; Allison 1972).

In recent years, cellular immunity to herpesvirus has been studied in vitro by using lymphocytes from immunized animals and man. Rosenberg et al. (1972) report on the in vitro transformation of immune rabbit lymphocytes by herpesvirus antigens and stress the value of this technique in assessing cell-mediated immunity. Wilton et al. (1972) investigated cell-mediated response to HVH type 1 in patients with primary and recurrent herpes-virus infection by employing techniques of macrophage migration inhibition, lymphocyte cytotoxicity and lymphocyte transformation. They found impaired macrophage migration inhibition and lymphocyte cytotoxicity in their patients with recurrent herpesvirus infection. However, lymphocyte transformation was not impaired in these patients. In the light of these findings they speculate that susceptibility to recurrences may be due to impaired production of migration inhibitory factor (MIF) and lymphotoxin (LT). In another recent study in patients with recurrent cold sores, Russell (1974) also found a normal lymphocyte transformation response to herpesvirus antigens.

Rasmussen et al. (1974) made a serial study of lymphocyte transformation and interferon production in individuals with HVH infection. Their results indicate intact lymphocyte transformation and increased interferon production in some individuals with oral herpetic lesions. They noted that herpes recurrences were more frequent in those subjects who failed to produce a detectable interferon response during or after the disease.

Perhaps the most comprehensive study of cellular immunity to herpes is that reported by Rosenberg and Notkins (1974) who investigated the immune responses to infectious and noninfectious virus in the rabbit. Their findings indicate that animals inoculated with infectious virus developed first cellular and then humoral immunity. Animals inoculated with ultraviolet-inactivated herpesvirus developed a cellular immune response but failed to develop humoral immunity, whereas animals inoculated with the virus complexed with specific antibody developed neither a cellular nor a humoral immune response. Moreover they showed that specifically sensitized lymphocytes could be stimulated in vitro by the virus and by virus-bearing cells, but not by infected cells that had been incubated with specific antiviral antibody. These observations lend further support to the current view that humoral antibodies can inhibit lymphocyte stimulation if they form complexes in antibody excess.

Evidently the situation in vivo is complex and the development of cell-mediated immunity may be influenced by a number of factors related to both the host and the antigen. It seems reasonable to conclude therefore, that cellular immunity should be studied by many approaches and not by a single method or reaction; it is a complex phenomenon and simplification could be misleading. In addition, studies concerning the immune response of the host to virus infections should also consider the possible effect of the virus itself on the function of the immune system (Notkins et al. 1970).

III Immunologic tissue injury in viral infections

Experimental findings strongly suggest that immune reactions which control many virus infections may contribute to the pathogenesis of tissue injury. In general, immune tissue damage can result either from cytotoxic reactions or from hypersensitivity reactions. Both can be mediated by circulating antibody or by sensitized lymphocytes. In cytotoxic reactions, antiviral antibody or sensitized lymphocytes or both interact with virus-induced cell surface antigens and damage the infected cells. In hypersensitivity reactions, the antibody reacts with antigens unrelated to those of the tissue and the resultant antigen-antibody complexes produce the injury. In many instances allergic reactions and inflammation result from the release of biologically active mediators.

Many reports have been published indicating that antiviral antibody and complement can injure virus-infected cells. Several years ago, Daniels et al. (1970) demonstrated that the interaction of antiserum to herpesvirus with herpesvirus antigens can activate the complement sequence. Brier et al. (1970) report a study indicating that herpesvirus infected cells release a chemotaxis-generating factor that cleaves the fifth component of complement. The product of this cleavage (C5a) is chemotactic for polymorphonuclear leukocytes and has anaphylatoxic properties (Shin et al. 1968; Jensen et al. 1969).

In another series of in vitro experiments, Brier et al. (1971) obtained evidence that herpesvirus can induce new antigens on the surface of various cells and that these cells become susceptible to the cytolytic effect of immune anti-HVH serum. Incubation of infected cells with specific antibody and complement resulted in cell damage within hours after incubation as measured by the release of radioactivity from Cr-labeled cells. In addition, they showed that cytolytic antibodies appeared in the serum of HVH infected rabbits almost simultaneously with the appearance of neutralizing antibody.

Using another experimental approach, Yang and Wentworth (1972) were also able to show that exposure of herpes virus infected cells to specific antiviral antibody and complement results in cell injury. In a more recent work, Yang et al. (1973) examined human sera for the presence of cytolytic activity against herpesvirus antigens. They found that sera positive for neutralizing activity also showed cytolytic activity, whereas sera negative for neutralizing activity failed to produce the cytotoxic effect. The cytotoxic activity of human sera on cells infected with either type 1 or type 2 HVH is clearly indicated also by the work of Smith et al. (1972a) who used the 51 Cr-technique.

Although these findings are very suggestive there is no direct evidence as yet that cytotoxic antibody is responsible for the production of herpes lesions in vivo. These antibodies may or may not have similar cytotoxic activity in vivo, but they surely deserve further study because of their potential pathogenic significance.

Cell-mediated immune response has also been implicated as a factor responsible, at least in part, for the pathologic effects observed during the course of herpesvirus infection. In 1966, Lausch *et al.* reported the development of delayed hypersensitivity to herpesvirus in guinea pigs sensitized by footpad injection of HVH in adjuvant. In studying the ocular response to herpesvirus these investigators observed that the maximum inflammatory response occurred 72 hours after intracorneal challenge in animals sensitized 3 days previously by footpad injection (Swyers *et al.* 1967).

More recently, Meyers and Pettit (1973) reported an extensive study demonstrating that the corneal response to herpesvirus antigens in sensitized guinea pigs paralleled the onset of the cutaneous delayed hypersensitivity reaction and of the in vitro inhibition of macrophage migration by the antigen at 7 days after sensitization. Moreover, they showed that the corneal clouding occurred before circulating antibodies to herpesvirus could be detected in the animals. These and similar observations (Chandler *et al.* 1971) strongly suggest that corneal inflammation in herpes keratitis could result from the release of soluble mediators by sensitized lymphocytes.

Although it is clear that we are only at the beginning of an understanding of the great complexity of the immune function, there is little doubt that a systematic approach to the manifold parameters of the immune system will ultimately lead to the resolution of many practical problems associated with various disease states.

Chapter 4

GENITAL HERPES

I Introduction

An interesting historical review of herpes genitalis has been presented by the English dermatologist Hutfield (1968). He credits Jean Astruc, a French physician, with the classical description of genital herpes, recorded in his book entitled *De morbis venereis* (1736), and quotes the first book on genital herpes, *Les herpes genitaux* by Diday and Doyon, published in 1886. These authors were the first to describe herpetic urethritis. The histology of genital herpetic vesicles was first recorded by Unna in 1898. Although the clinical features of herpes genitalis were recognized and described more than 200 yers ago, the causative agent of this clinical entity was not identified until 1946 when Slavin and Gavett isolated herpesvirus from vulvar lesions. Several years later, herpesvirus was isolated from the male genital tract (Duxbury and Lawrence 1959).

Nevertheless, rapid advance in this area has only come within recent years. Interest in genital herpetic infections has been revived by recent findings indicating that herpesvirus (HVH) isolated from genital lesions differs antigenically and biologicallv from HVH's that commonly infect nongenital sites of the body (Schneweis 1962; Dowdle *et al.* 1967). According to the ingenious classification of Nahmias (1972), the grea⁺ majority of HVH strains recovered from the human body above the waist belong to type 1, whereas the great majority from sites below the waist belong to type 2. Experimental studies have also suggested that type 2 HVH has a special genitotropism (Nahmias *et al.* 1967c, 1971b; London *et al.* 1971; Felsburg *et al.* 1972). Since it has been realized that the external genitalia are not the only site of infection but that deeper genital tissues such as the cervix, may be invaded by herpetic infection also, the term "herpes progenitalis" is no longer adequate (Nahmias 1972).

In recent years it has become clear that genital herpes in the mother may be the major, although not the only source of virus for the newborn. In addition the possible association between genital herpes and cervical carcinoma has been suggested by studies conducted independently by three groups of investigators working in Atlanta (Nahmias *et al.*), in Houston (Melnick *et al.*), and in Baltimore (Aurelian *et al.*).

All these considerations have given a strong impetus to research on herpetic infections during the last few years (Kawana *et al.* 1976).

II Incidence

The frequency of clinically manifest primary and recurrent genital herpetic infections is difficult to assess. Early clinical studies conducted in Hamburg by Unna (1883) indicated an incidence of approximately 8 percent among female and 1 percent among male patients attending venereal disease clinics. It is of interest that Nahmias *et al.* (1969a) reports an almost identical rate of clinically diagnosed genital herpes: 8 percent in females and of 0.5 percent in males. However, the rate of virologically confirmed cases was slightly lower: 6 percent in females and 0.3 percent in males.

A somewhat different incidence of genital herpes (8 percent in females and 5.4 percent in males) was found by Jeansson and Molin (1971) in Sweden in a study of patients attending a venereal disease department. In contrast, the general population had an incidence of 0.5 percent among females and 0.0 percent in a small group of healthy young males. However Kleger *et al.* (1968) reported lower incidence of genital herpes in a female population at risk (1.6 percent) as compared to the general population (0.1 per cent). On the other hand the prevalence of herpesvirus in the genital secretions of the prostitute population was 6.9 percent (Duenas *et al.* 1972). It appears that the incidence of genital herpes varies from 1.6 to 8 percent in females at risk, and from 0.3 to 5.4 percent in the corresponding male population.

These data indicate that genital herpes is not a rare infection in humans. According to estimates by Nahmias there may be around 200 000 cases of genital herpes in the United States each year, of which one quarter to one third are primary infections (Josey 1973).

Epidemiologic surveys in patients with clinically evident genital herpes or in patients with other venereal diseases cannot yield reliable estimates of the incidence of genital herpes infection.

Recognition that many cases of genital herpes may be asymptomatic, along with improved cytologic and virologic diagnosis, has led to more reliable estimates (Poste *et al.* 1972). Apparently, more accurate data have been obtained from surveys in women undergoing routine *cervical cytology examinations* (Wilbanks *et al.* 1970). Papanicolaou smears of the cervix are particularly helpful in detecting subclinical herpetic cervicitis in women (Nahmias and Josey, 1976). In such surveys typical herpetic cytologic changes were found in 0.03 to 0.5 percent of the women examined (Nahmias *et al.* 1969a; Wolinska and Melamed 1970; Naib 1966; Kleger *et al.* 1968; An 1969). The two largest series are presented by Wolinska and Melamed (43 331 women), and by Nahmias *et al.* (91 845 women). In the former the incidence of herpetic cytologic changes was 0.09 percent, whereas in the series reported by Nahmias *et al.* it was 0.48 percent. These rates are within the ranges obtained for the general population. Cytologic changes (nuclear inclusion bodies) suggesting herpetic infection were much higher in vaginal smears from patients with vaginal discharge than those found in routine smears; 11 percent in a study by Cederqvist *et al.* (1970).

The role of socioeconomic factors in determining the rate of genital herpes was first recognized by Unna (1883). In recent years considerable evidence has accumulated showing the importance of these factors (Beilby *et al.* 1968; Rawls *et al.* 1968b, 1969). Epidemiologic surveys by Kleger *et al.* (1968). and Ng *et al.* 1970a,b have clearly shown a greater prevalence of genital herpesvirus infection among women of lower income classes. This has been confirmed by serological studies conducted in Houston (Rawls *et al.* 1970a, b, 1971; Kaufman and Melnick 1971).

Because of the probable venereal mode of transmission, genital herpes is often found in association with other venereal diseases. In contrast to a high incidence of genital herpes infection among sexually promiscuous women, nuns were found to be virtually free of this disease (Nahmias *et al.*, 1970c).

Little is known about the *long term incidence* of type 2 HVH infections in humans. A large percentage of asymptomatic primary infections together with the appearance of lesions on sites that are not readily accessible (cervix, urethra) makes precise analysis even more difficult. In an ideal prospective study Nahmias *et al.* (1973b) suggest that the annual rate of primary infection with type 2 HVH could be approximately 3 percent in women over 20 years of age and low socioeconomic status.

There is also evidence indicating that genital herpes is more frequent in *pregnant women* than in gynecological patients (Ng *et al.* 1970b; Nahmias *et al.* 1971). It might be that the virus persists longer in the genital tract of pregnant women or that gravidae are more regularly examined. The possibility of hormonal influence should also be considered. Because of the possible effect on the fetus, genital herpes in pregnancy deserves particular attention.

The presence of recurrent herpes immediately prior to menstruation might be related to a change in hormonal levels leading to an increased susceptibility to genital herpes (Poste *et al.* 1972).

The incidence of genital herpes appears to be lower among persons using mechanical (condom) prophylaxis (Poste *et al.* 1972). In this connection the question has arisen as to whether the use of contraceptive drugs, which permits greater liberty in sexual contacts, could be responsible for a higher rate of genital herpes.

Genital herpes in males has been described by Astruc and several other workers. From the available data it appears that clinically overt genital herpes is not encountered in males as frequently as in females (Sorice 1971). The literature concerning genital herpes in males is scarce (Barile *et al.* 1962; Parker and Banatvala 1967). At present it is not clear whether the reason for this lies in diagnostic difficulties or in incompleteness of routine examinations in males.

Information regarding the incidence of antibodies to type 2 herpesvirus is mainly derived from serologic surveys that have been made among males. Nervetheless, it does not seem very likely that in the transmission of genital herpes the male does not have a significant role. It has been proposed that the male genital tract might be the major reservoir for type 2 herpesvirus (Centifanto *et al.* 1972). Obviously this subject requires further epidemiologic study.

III Serology

Concepts regarding the natural course of genital herpes infections have changed radically within recent years. Although genital herpes is rare in children it is frequently encountered in adults. Since the great majority (70—90) percent of adults have been found to possess neutralizing antibodies to herpesvirus, cases of genital herpes were considered to represent recurrent attacks (Hutfield 1968). However, with the recognition of type 2 HVH this concept has been revised. It is evident now that antibodies to type 1 HVH do not protect against type 2 HVH and vice versa. Normally infection with type 1 HVH occurs before that with type 2 HVH. Primary infection with type 2 HVH usually appears later in life when sexual activity begins. Antibodies produced in response to type 1 HVH have been shown to neutralize type 1 more efficiently than type 2 viruses. Infection with type 2 HVH induces antibodies that neutralize type 2 HVH slightly better than type 1 HVH (Plummer *et al.* 1970; Rawls *et al.* 1971).

Type 2 HVH ("genital type") is the predominant cause of genital herpes, but in certain cases genital herpes may be caused by type 1 HVH. The rate at which type 1 HVH participates in the etiology of genital herpes varies from 5 to 13.5 percent (Nahmias *et al.* 1970; Nahmias and Roizman 1973a, b; Kaufman *et al.* 1973a). The higher rates are not well documented.

Type 1 HVH appears to be a common etiologic agent of genital herpes in children who have had no sexual contact. However, in children who have had sexual contacts type 2 HVH is the predominant infection agent (Nahmias *et al.* 1968). The rise in the serum antibody titers in the reconvalescent phase is firm evidence of a primary infection with herpesvirus. The occurrence of clinically evident genital herpes in patients with high titers of neutralizing antibodies is considered to represent a recurrent attack.

Primary infection in the etiology of genital herpes is estimated at from one fourth to one third of all patients (Ng *et al.* 1970a,b; Nahmias *et al.* 1969a; Josey 1973).

With the development of new concepts regarding primary and recurrent herpetic infections the older terminology is no longer accurate. For instance, there is the problem of how to designate a case of recurrent type 1 HVH infection with concomitant type 2 HVH infection.

In an attempt to establish a more adequate nomenclature, Nahmias has proposed a classification (Table 1) based on the type of antibodies present in the serum and type of HVH isolated.

Table 1. *Classification of herpetic infection* (*Nahmias* 1972, modified by M. Juretić)

Antibody type at beginning	Virus type recovered	Infection	Antibody type at end
None present	1	Primary 1	1
None present	2	Primary 2	2
1	2	Primary 2	1 and 2
2	1	Primary 1	1 and 2
1	1	Recurrent 1	1
2	2	Recurrent 2	2
1 and 2	1	Recurrent 1	1 and 2
1 and 2	2	Recurrent 2	1 and 2

Therefore, morbidity of HVH-1 and HVH-2 in a study population may result in no evident infection or in primary HVH-1 or HVH-2 infection but without recurrences with either virus. The other epidemiological variations are a recurrent infection with one HVH type only or a recurrent infection with one type and a first infection with the other type, and recurrent infections with both HVH-1 and HVH-2 (Nahmias and Josey, 1976).

Infections with type 2 HVH occasionally occur at nongenital sites of the body. For instance, the fingers may be involved more frequently than the mouth. The anal region and the thighs may also be the site of type 2 HVH infections. Herpetic infection of the anus, resulting from unusual sexual contact (homosexuality) is probably caused by the same virus type although there is a lack of more detailed information about such cases.

The available serologic data indicate that *infection with type 2 HVH in humans depends on age, socioeconomic status and frequency of sexual intercourse.* Data presented by Nahmias indicate that antibodies to type 1 HVH are present in approximately 70 percent of the adult female population. The remaining 30 percent have either dual or type 2 specific neutralizing antibodies. This information is derived from surveys conducted in adult females of low income class. The influence of economic factors is also revealed by the studies of Rawls which show that antibodies to type 2 HVH are present in about 9 percent of women from the higher socioeconomic groups, and in about 22 percent of women from the lower income class. Among prostitutes this frequency is much higher, from 54 percent (Rawls *et al.* 1970a) to 100 percent. Duenas *et al.* (1972) report the occurrence of antibodies against HVH type 2 in from 65 to 73 percent of prostitutes over 20 years of age. The frequency of antibodies was dependent on present age and the duration of prostitution but was not related to racial differences. However in a survey series of 35 nuns, reported by Nahmias *et al.* (1970b), only one had type 2 neutralizing antibodies.

The frequency of antibodies to type 2 HVH as reported by other investigators varied from 18 percent among women of higher socioeconomic status (Plummer and Masterson 1971) to 55 percent among low-income black women (Royston and Aurelian 1970).

The prevalence of antibodies to both types of herpesvirus is clearly correlated with and similarly influenced by annual income and living conditions (McDonald *et al.* 1974a).

The dynamics of antibody appearance from birth to adulthood is illustrated in Fig. 8. Antibodies to either type 1 or type 2 HVH possessed by the mother are transferred to the fetus across the placenta. They decline during the first 6 months of postnatal life. Type 2 specific antibodies usually begin to appear in females

46

after the age of 14 years. The final rate of these antibodies in the adult female population varies from 20 to 60 percent among those of lower, and from 10 to 20 percent among those of higher socio-economic classes. In certain groups of the population these differences are even more marked. In the adult male population extensive sero-epidemiologic surveys have not been made.

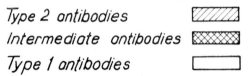

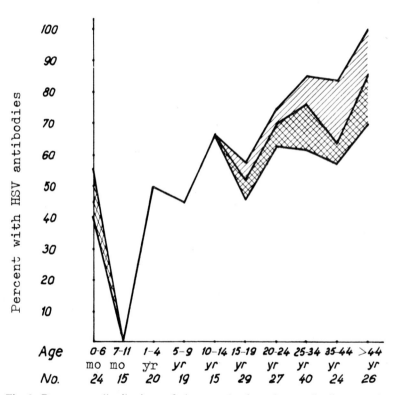

Fig. 8. Percentage distribution of herpes simplex virus antibodies type 1, type 2, and intermediate (type 1 + type 2) in 239 individuals of varying age groups (Nahmias *et al.* 1970 b).

The pattern of antibodies against HVH type 2 according to age in a seroepidemiologic study in Japan (Sawanobori 1973), was congruent with other data presented here.

The role of recurrent herpetic infections in maintaining a constant level of HVH antibodies over long periods is not yet entirely clear.

IV Age and sex distribution

The age distribution of primary genital herpes can be estimated from serologic data, though isolation of the virus is more difficult in males than in females (Nahmias *et al.* 1969a).

The highest rate of genital herpes in women is found in the younger age group, among teenagers (Nahmias *et al.*, 1969a). In the series presented by Ng *et al.* (1970b), the highest rate was found in the group of mean age 26.4 years. The entire age distribution is illustrated in Fig. 9. In another survey, the mean age of women with primary genital herpes was 26.6 years, whereas the mean age of women with recurrent infection was 36.5 years (Rawls *et al.* 1971).

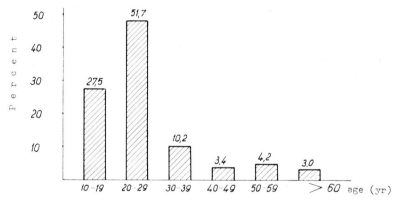

Fig. 9. Age distribution of 256 women with symptomatic (53.2 percent) or asymptomatic (46.8 percent) genital herpes (Ng *et al.* 1970 b).

A similar age distribution has been found in other studies of women attending centers for family planning (Wolinska and Melamed 1970; Masukawa *et al.* 1972). This is shown in Fig. 10.

Although the age distribution and natural course of genital herpes in males has received only little attention, there is no reason to believe that in this regard males differ from females. In a series

48

presented by Parker and Banatvala (1967) the ages of 21 males with clinically evident genital herpes ranged from 20 to 42 years, the mean age being 29 years. The most probable reason for such a high mean age is the fact that the series included patients with recurrent genital herpes.

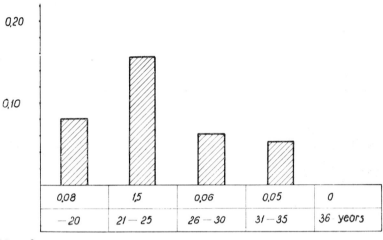

No. of

women   6   22   6   3

Fig. 10 Age distribution of 37 women with cytologic evidence of herpes. The rate is given as the percentage of 43 331 females in the general population (Wolinska and Melamed 1970).

Seasonal variations in the occurrence of genital herpes do not seem to be significant, though a summer peak was noted in one of the studies (Masukawa *et al.* 1972).

V Transmission and incubation

The possibility that genital herpes could be transmitted venereally was recognized early in the history of this disease. In 1923 Lipschütz named the disease "Koituskrankheit."

Genital herpes is a disease that predominates in the adult population. This is revealed by clinical experience and serologic surveys. Hence, the earlier concept that it represents a recurrent form of primary infection acquired in childhood has long been abandoned (Krugman 1952; Lazar 1955; Yen *et al.* 1965).

There is now abundant evidence that the infection is acquired by sexual contact with an infected partner (Sharlit 1940; Slavin and Gavett, 1946; Lazar 1955; Duxbury and Lawrence 1959). In the series reported by Barile *et al.* (1962), herpesvirus proved to be the most common cause of penile lesions among U. S. armed forces personnel in Japan. The patients examined were young, had contacts with prostitutes, and the great majority of them neglected the use of prophylaxis. Finally, Nahmias *et al.* (1969a) has characterized genital herpes as a *"commonly occurring venereal disease."* Genital herpetic infection appeared in seven out of eight females who had contact with males with penile herpes. An *attack rate* similar to this was reported by Rawls *et al.* (1971), who found HVH type 2 infection in 14 out of 18 contacts (78 percent) of men with genital herpes.

The significantly higher incidence of genital herpes among prostitutes and patients attending venereal disease clinics, and the fact that children are practically free from genital herpes infections, indicates that *venereal transmission is the most important mechanism spreading the virus in the human population* (Nahmias and Hutton 1972; Adam *et al.* 1972). It also seems apparent that early heterosexual activity favors the occurrence of HVH type 2 neutralizing antibodies early in life (Josey *et al.* 1966): antibodies do not appear in the population until the age when heterosexual activity begins.

The available evidence indicates that the frequency of genital herpes is significantly higher among women attending antivenereal clinics than among those receiving routine cervical examinations (Beilby *et al.* 1968; Kleger *et al.* 1968; Rawls *et al.* 1971). Indeed, genital herpes was frequently found in association with other venereal disease (Barile *et al.* 1962; Nahmias *et al.* 1973a).

The venereal mode of transmission has also been demonstrated in experimental animals, including rabbits (Levaditi 1926), mice (Nahmias *et al.* 1967c) and monkeys (Nahmias *et al.* 1971b; London *et al.* 1971; Felsburg *et al.* 1972; Kalter *et al.* 1972).

Although genital herpes is rare in children it may nevertheless result from either venereal or nonvenereal transmission (Legendre 1953; Nahmias *et al.* 1968). It is possible that 5 to 10 percent of genital herpes may be due to type 1 HVH (Nahmias 1972). However, in such cases extragenital sites of the body (fingers, mouth) are usually affected by the infection as well (Slavin and Gavett, 1946; Krugman 1942). But it has been observed that type 2 HVH infections can occasionally affect nongenital sites of the body, including the perianal region (Sheward 1961; Hutfield 1968), pubic region and fingers (Parker and Banatvala 1967), and the thighs and pharynx (Kaufman and Rawls 1972, Kaufman *et al.* 1973a).

The transmission of HVH infection by orogenital sexual contact is frequently the result of type 1 (Hutton and Stegman 1973). The genitooral mode of transmission is, on the other hand, associated with HVH type 2 infection (Kaufman *et al.* 1973a).

At present it is not entirely clear whether reinfection with the homologous virus type can also occur. Earlier work showed that herpetic lesions may be experimentally produced at different sites, usually on the skin. More recently Nahmias *et al.* (1967c) reported the successful reinfection of mice and monkeys with the homologous type 2 HVH.

The incubation period of type 1 herpetic infection has been shown to be 2 to 12 days with a mean of 6 days (Juretić 1960). In type 2 infections an incubation period of from 2 to 7 days has been reported by several investigators (Sharlit 1950; Barile *et al.* 1962). Experiments on animals have also indicated that clinical symptoms of the infection appear after an incubation period of 5 to 7 days (London *et al.* 1971; Felsburg *et al.* 1972; Kalter *et al.* 1972).

A case report of extragenital type 2 infection occuring after orogenital contact indicates that oral lesions appeared after an incubation period of 3 days whereas vulvar lesions occurred after 5 days (Kaufman and Rawls 1972). Probably the incubation period does not depend only on the type of virus inoculated. Catalano reports the observation of an incubation period of exactly 4 days in consorts (cited by London *et al.* 1971).

On the basis of these data it appears *the incubation period of genital* HVH *infection varies from 2 to 7 days with a mean of 5 days.*

The source of type 2 HVH infection has not yet been elucidated. Epidemiologically, all carriers of the virus, whether their infections are symptomatic or asymptomatic, are equally important. It is known that genital herpetic infections are more prone to recur than nongenital infections. The rate of asymptomatic carriers of type 2 HVH is not known, but it probably varies with age, socioeconomic status, profession and frequency of sexual intercourse with different partners. It probably also depends on many other factors such as the mode and time of specimen collection and the analysis of the specimen.

Obviously, the rate of positive type 2 HVH findings in suspected cases, that is in a selected population is high. Ng *et al.* (1970b) report that approximately one half of the women in their series were asymptomatic at the time herpes genitalis was detected. However, in the general population the rate of herpes genitalis appears to be significantly lower. For example, by examining approximately 67 000 cytologic specimens from about 43 300 women attending the Centers for Planned Parenthood of New York City, Wolinska and Melamed (1970) found evidence of herpes genitalis at an overall rate of 0.09 percent. These and similar data reported from other centers (Centifanto *et al.* 1971), indicate a low rate of asymptomatic genital carriers of type 2 HVH in a female population. On the other hand, in a series of 190 randomly selected male patients of various age groups, Centifanto *et al.* found an incidence of 15 percent positive for herpesvirus type 2. It is of interest that specimens collected from the prostate and vas deferens gave a higher percentage of positives than did specimens collected from other sites of the genitourinary tract, including urethral swabs, testicular biopsies and foreskin tissues. These findings have been interpreted as indicating that *the male genitourinary tract is a reservoir for the genital strain of herpesvirus.* The high incidence of virus isolates from deeper parts of the genitourinary tract suggest that such a reservoir may be analogous to the reservoir of HVH in the lacrimal gland. Certainly further study is required for the elucidation of this subject.

However, aside from the question of where the main reservoir of the virus is there seems to be no doubt that genital herpesvirus infection is a venereal disease which goes back and forth between the male and female like a ping-pong ball.

VI Clinical features

A. *In females*

Clinical feature of genital herpesvirus infections do not differ significantly from those seen in extragenital infections. A summary of clinical symptoms associated with genital herpes as published by Ng *et al.* (1970) is presented in Tables 2—4.

Table 2. *Symptoms associated with herpes genitalis in 252 women* (Ng *et al.* 1970).

Symptoms	Patients	
	Number	Percent
Asymptomatic	118	46.8
Constitutional	37	14.7
Vaginal discharge	92	36.5
Genital pain	88	34.9
Dysuria	21	8.3
Vaginal bleeding	8	3.2

4*

Table 3. *Lesions indicative of herpes genitalis* (Ng *et al.* 1970b).

Lesions	Number	Percent
None	105	41.7
Ulceration	129	51.2
Vesicles	24	9.5
Papules	20	7.9
Lymphadenopathy	19	7.5

Table 4. *Location of lesions in women with herpes genitalis* (Ng *et al.* 1970b).

Location	Lesions	
	Number	Percent
Vulva	102	40.5
Cervix	58	23.0
Vagina	38	15.1
Perineum	9	3.6
Thigh	2	0.8

Primary herpetic infection is usually accompanied by clinical symptoms such as fever, pain, dysuria, vaginal discharge and inguinal lymphadenopathy. The lesions involve the labia majora and the vestibule of the vulva, vagina and cervix (Poste *et al.* 1972).

The occurrence of genital herpes immediately before and during menstruation ("herpes catameniale") appears to be the result more of a recurrent attack than of the primary infection (Hutfield 1968).

Primary infection with genital herpesvirus seems to be less severe in individuals with type 1 HVH neutralizing antibodies than in individuals without HVH antibodies (Rawls *et al.* 1971; Kaufman *et al.* 1973a). Herpetic lesions that develop during the course of primary infection usually persist for a long time (Kaufman *et al.* 1973a). Good correlation was found between the clinical impression and the laboratory diagnosis of the primary or the recurrent disease.

Until recently vulvovaginitis was considered to be the dominant clinical symptom of genital herpes. However, cytologic examinations have revealed typical herpetic inclusions in the uterine cervix (Stern and Longo 1963). The first case of an isolated herpetic cervicitis was described by Nigogosyan and Mills (1965). Following this observation herpesvirus infection of the cervix has been reported with increasing frequency (Yen *et al.* 1965; Stcin and Siciliano 1966). Usually the affected cervix is erythematous and edematous, a diffuse cervicitis develops with the appearance of ulcerations; vesicles develop rarely. However, cases with severe necrotic lesions resembling malignant changes have also been described (Wilcox 1968; Stein and Siciliano 1966). The available data indicate that the rate of cervical involvement in genital herpes varies from 23 percent to 65 percent (Ng *et al.* 1970b; Josey *et al.* 1966). Still, asymptomatic herpesvirus infections of the cervix and vagina are more frequent than asymptomatic infections of the vulva. It seems that asymptomatic infections are important as they allow uncontrolled transmission of the virus. Asymptomatic forms of genital herpes appear to be more frequent in recurrent infections. The extent to which primary infection displays itself clinically is not known. Also, the factors leading to the manifestation of infection are far from clear.

Dysuria and the resulting urinary retention may develop in certain cases, so that endourethral lesions can also occur. Although some earlier observations suggested that herpetic infection may involve the urinary bladder, cytologic, virologic and serologic evidence has been obtained only recently (Masukawa *et al.* 1972; Person *et al.* 1973).

A case of herpetic involvement of the endometrium has been reported by Goldman (1970). However, virologic and serologic data that would confirm the diagnosis are lacking.

Genital herpes in women is frequently associated with other genital infections resulting from *Trichomonas vaginalis, Candida albicans, Haemophylus vaginalis and gonococci* (Kleger *et al.* 1968; Beilby *et al.* 1968).

Complications resulting from an attack of genital herpes have been described in the older literature as reviewed by Hutfield (1966).

B. *In males*

The basic morphologic characteristics of herpetic eruptions including erythema, papules, vesicles and ulcers are typical of genital herpes in males (Hutfield 1968). The lesions appear predominantly on the glans penis, prepuce and preputial sulcus, but may also occur on the shaft of the penis and on the scrotum.

Herpetic lesions of the perianal region and anus usually result from homosexual contacts (Hutfield 1968). Duxbury and Lawrence (1959) were the first to isolate herpesvirus from the male genitalia.

Complications resulting from genital herpes in males are not uncommon and usually include edema, balanoposthitis (Sorice 1971), phimosis and urethral strictures (Hutfield 1968).

From the relatively scant data reported in the literature it appears that the rate of genital herpes in males is higher among those with frequent sexual intercourse, particularly those who neglect the use of prophylaxis and those who are uncircumcised (Barile *et al.* 1962; Parker and Banatvala 1967).

Diday and Doyon (1876) in (cit. by Hutfield, 1966) first drew attention to the occurrence of urethral discharge and stinging on micturition in patients with genital herpes. Endourethral herpes is undoubtedly one of the many causes of nonspecific urethritis. The earlier literature contains several reports concerning herpetic urethritis in males. Yet Nasemann and Nagai (1960) were the first to report cases of urethritis with virologic evidence of herpesvirus as the causative agent.

Since the rate of herpetic infection of the male urethra is relatively high (0.3 percent according to Nahmias *et al.* 1969a and 4.2 percent according to Jeansson and Molin 1971), virologic tests should be conducted on every patient presenting urethral discharge. The value of this procedure is emphasized by the data reported by Centifanto *et al.* (1972) who indicated an incidence of 15 percent positive HVH cultures from specimens obtained not only from the urethra but also from the prostate and vas deferens.

The findings of Morrisseau *et al.* (1970) suggest an etiologic relation between herpes simplex virus and acute, nonbacterial prostatitis: of 12 patients with prostatitis 2 yielded HVH, and cytopathologic changes suggestive of HVH were noted in 4 others.

That neurologic complications (aseptic meningitis, myelitis, radiculitis or neuralgia) may arise as a result of genital herpes was recognized by early workers dealing with the subject (Gillot *et al.* 1958; Duxbury and Lawrence 1959). However, the mechanism by which HVH produces these disturbances is not yet clear. Cerebrospinal fluid from such patients usually shows pleocytosis but no other abnormalities (Nahmias and Roizman 1973).

C. *In children*

Genital herpes is rare among children. The first reported case, occurring in a molested girl, was described by Legendre in 1853 (cit. by Nahmias *et al.* 1968). Thereafter some sporadic cases were reported (Krugman 1952, Lazar, 1955). It is interesting to note that one out of three girls with primary genital infection presented by Scott et al. (1952) had a history of primary oral herpes.

More recently, Nahmias et al. (1968), reported their observations on six cases (five girls and boy) with genital herpes. Type 1 HVH was recovered from two and type 2 HVH from three of the six cases. The data on the boy suggested a reinfection with type 1. He had a previous clinical history of oral herpes and neutralizing antibodies were present in his serum during the acute phase. HVH type 1 was recovered from the penile lesions as well as from the mouth. In one of the girls genital herpes was associated with gingivostomatitis. In this case no history of venereal contact was obtained and the hymen ring was intact. These cases suggest that the virus can be transmitted from one to another site of the body. Clinical and laboratory data on the four other girls indicated a primary type 2 HVH infection. Although the infection was most probably acquired by sexual contact in all four of them, only two gave histories of such contact.

Discussing this subject, the authors emphasize the importance of follow-up of children with genital herpes throughout adulthood because of the possible association of such infection with pregnancy and with certain other diseases.

Genital infection with HVH type 1 and 2 in children is a problem that requires further investigation.

VII Prenatal herpes

Herpes virus infections appear to be more frequent among pregnant women than in the general female population (Ng et al. 1970b).

Earlier sero-epidemiologic surveys of pregnant women revealed a rate of 2.5 percent (Sever and White 1968). However, more recent serologic studies have indicated a signifiicantly lower rate. Thus in a study of 4 930 gravida Korones et al. (1970) found seroconversion to HVH in only 0.3 percent. In another prospective survey conducted by Nahmias et al. (1971a,c) the incidence of herpesvirus infection among pregnant women was found to be 1.02 percent. This value is twice that obtained from a general control population. The influence of hormones has not been determined.

Maternal herpetic infection during gestation may affect the fetus in several different ways and result in *congenital malformations, abortion, stillbirth and prematurity or constitutional disease of the fetus and the newborn.* Congenital malformations and abortion occur during early pregnancy. A transplacental hematogenic path of infection is considered to be the exclusive sibility.

Congenital anomalies subsequent to herpetic infection have been published in a very few cases. The most frequent anomalies are shown in Table 6. All reported cases were etiologically associated with HVH type 2 infections, except one case published by Florman *et al.* (1973) in which intranuclear eosinophilic inclusions were found in the urine sediment.

Table 5. *Congenital malformations with intrauterine acquired herpesvirus infections*

	Sch..ffer and Avery (1965)	South et al. (1969)	Mur-phy[+] (1970)	Rubio[+] (1970)	Alford[+] (1970)	Florman et al. (1973)
Microcephaly	+	+	—	—	+	—
Intracranial calcifications	+	+	—	—	—	+
Diffuse brain damage	—	+	+	—	+	+
Chorioretinitis	—	—	+	+	—	—
Retinal dysplasia	—	+	—	—	—	—
Microophthalmia	+	—	—	—	—	—
Vesicular rath	At birth	At birth	At birth	Shortly after birth	Shortly after birth	None
Type of herpes virus	2	2	2	2	2	1

[+]Cited in Nahmias *et al.* (1970a).

Recently published data also suggest a causal relation between herpesvirus infection and fetal malformation. In a prospective study during and after pregnancy, 224 mothers were tested for antibodies against ten different viruses. The excess in the defective group was mainly due to high antibody titers against herpesvirus types 1 and 2, cytomegalovirus and varicella-zoster (Lapinleimu *et al.* 1974).

The group of investigators working in Atlanta (Naib *et al.* 1970) has clearly indicated an association between maternal genital herpetic infection and spontaneous *abortion.* In 283 women with genital herpes detected during the first 20 weeks of gestation,

34 percent of the pregnanices terminated in abortion. This rate is three times that in uninfected gravida (10%). The results obtained from a smaller study group showed a significantly higher abortion rate (54%) among gravida with primary genital herpes. In a study of spontaneous abortion, Bouè and Loffredo (1970) isolated HVH type 2 from the embryonic tissue.

The pathogenic mechanism for fetal damage due to herpesvirus infection involves *transplacental transfer of the virus to the fetus*. That herpesvirus can be transmitted across the placenta was first recognized by Zuelzer and Stulberg (1952) who found primary herpetic infection in a newborn delivered by cesarean section. The presence of clinically evident herpetic infection in infants at birth strongly suggests that the infection is acquired prenatally. This view is strengthened by the fact that infections acquired during delivery or postnatally require a minimal incubation period of 2 to 3 days. There have been several reports of neonatal herpes with the disease clinically evident at the time of birth (Michell and MacCallum 1963; Sieber *et al.* 1966; Nahmias 1967a, b; Torphy *et al.* 1970; Pettay *et al.* 1972). From a recent analysis of 85 cases of neonatal herpes it appears that in 14 percent of them the disease occurred within the first 48 hours after birth (Sorice 1971).

Placental lesions observed in association with neonatal herpes infection lend further support to the concept that herpesvirus infection may be transplacentally transmitted (Witzleben and Driscoll 1965; Guha *et al.* 1968; Sieber *et al.* 1966; Altshuler 1974). Earlier studies on rabbits have also provided evidence for transplacental infection with herpes virus (Biegeleisen and Scott 1958; Middelkamp *et al.* 1967).

The analogy with other strains of herpes virus that are pathogenic for animals (equine, canine and feline) is very convincing. All these viruses affect the fetus across the placenta (Poste and King 1971).

Still another argument in favor of the transplacental transmission of herpesvirus in humans is the finding of elevated levels of immunoglobulin M (IgM) in the umbilical cord serum in the presence of intrauterine herpetic infection (Sieber *et al.* 1966; Sever and White 1968; Alford *et al.* 1969): elevated IgM in the cord serum is considered to be a sign of fetal production of macroglobulin antibodies in response to intrauterine infection.

Interesting observations regarding the association between maternal genital herpes and *prematurity* have been reported by Nahmias *et al.* (1971a). They suggest that the rate of premature birth is higher the later the mother develops genital herpetic infection in pregnancy. Thus the prematurity rate among women with genital herpes occurring during the first few weeks of pregnancy was found to be 16 percent, similar to the rate in the control population. However, when the infection occurred later during pregnancy the prematurity rate increased up to 30 percent. Moreover, it appears that this rate is even higher (35 percent) in the presence of primary infection.

Although studies in humans and in experimental animals suggest the transfer of herpesvirus across the placenta, other routes of virus transmission cannot be neglected. Apparently the fetus can be infected by an ascending route, particularly in mothers with asymptomatic or latent genital herpes. Early rupture of the membranes resulting from vaginal obstetric manipulation may also facilitate the ascending route of infection.

The most cogent *arguments for intrauterine herpetic infection* have been summarized by Sorice (1971) as follows:

(1) neonatal herpes present at the time of birth (Mitchell and McCallum 1963);
(2) the presence of neonatal herpes in infants delivered by cesarean section (Zuelzer and Stulberg 1952);
(3) recovery of virus from the umbilical cord and the placenta (Gagnon, 1968; Patrizi *et al.* 1968);
(4) the presence of typical placental lesions (Witzleben and Driscoll 1965);
(5) increased levels of IgM in cord serum (Sieber *et al.* 1966);
(6) the six reported cases of congenital malformations due to herpes virus infection (Florman *et al.* 1973);
(7) experimental evidence of transplacental transmission of herpesvirus (Biegeleisen and Scott 1958);
(8) the findings that primary genital herpes increases the rates of abortion and prematurity (Nahmias *et al.* 1971a).

Herpesvirus can be isolated from apparently healthy newborns (Sanders and Cramblett 1968). Although primary herpetic infection in the newborn is usually fatal, milder forms also occur. However, it has been observed that a mild herpetic infection in the newborn results later in severe psychomotor retardation (Hovig *et al.* 1968). This raises the question whether asymptomatic or subclinical herpesvirus infection of the fetus and newborn can lead to various injuries later in life (Poste *et al.* 1972).

In a prospective survey Korones *et al.* found 18 gravida who showed serologic evidence of genital herpes infection but only one of their infants developed herpesvirus infection. The other

17 offspring showed no sign of the infection during a four-year period of observation. The reason for this may well lie in the fact that the study covered gravida in whom seroconversion occurred mostly after the first trimester of pregnancy.

An interesting case report by Rekant (1973) shows that eczema herpeticum during pregnancy may also be without consequences for the developing fetus.

Obviously, genital herpes of the mother may sometimes, but not always, affect the developing fetus. Fetal affection probably depends upon the time of acquisition of herpesvirus, the amount of virus inoculated and many other still poorly defined factors. Therefore, further prospective surveys are required in order to evaluate exactly the risk of herpes infection for the fetus.

Chapter 5

NEONATAL HERPES

I Introduction

The first case of neonatal herpes appearing in the form of conjunctivitis was reported in 1934 by Batignani, an Italian ophthalmologist. At that time neonatal herpes was thought to be a rare disease. It was believed that passively acquired maternal antibodies were efficient in protecting the fetus and newborn from infection with herpesvirus. The suspicion that HVH might be responsible for severe neonatal infection was first expressed by the American pathologist Hass in 1935. On postmortem examination of a premature infant he found intranuclear inclusion bodies and necrosis in the parenchymal cells of the liver and the adrenal glands. Several years later, Smith *et al.* (1941) isolated herpesvirus from the brain tissue of an infant who died of encephalitis. Thereafter, Quilligan and Wilson (1951) and Florman and Mindlin (1952) recovered the virus from skin lesions and liver of neonates who died with signs of sepsis. A particular susceptibility of very young organisms to infection with HVH is evident also from studies in experimental animals (Anderson 1940, Kilbourne and Horsfall 1951).

Between 1951 and 1963 approximately 50 cases of neonatal herpes were reported. Zuelzer and Stulberg (1952) were the first to describe disseminated herpetic infection in older infants. It has become apparent that prematures and twins are particularly susceptible to HVH infection (France and Wilmers 1953, Zuelzer and Stulberg 1952, Florman and Mindlin 1952; In the published case reports, the disease always had a sudden onset and a septic course. The patients survived but usually with severe neurologic sequelae (Florman and Mindlin 1952. Epstein and Crouch 1954). The favorable outcome of one neonate with herpes virus infection was first reported in France in 1930 (Lamy *et al.* 1960; Bach *et al.,* 1960).

Clinical features and pathologic findings have been repeatedly described by numerous authors working in the United States

(McDougal *et al.* 1954, Brain 1956, Clark 1965), in France (Le Tan Vinh *et al.* 1955, Neimann *et al.* 1963, Mozziconacci *et al.* 1955), in Australia (Williams and Jack, 1955, Colebatch 1955, Jack and Perry 1959), in the Nordic countries (Ericsson *et al.* 1958, Langvad and Voigt 1963, Szogi and Berge 1966, Vluge *et al.* 1967), in Czechoslovakia (Vortel and Herout 1957), in Switzerland (Felder *et al.* 1960) and in Japan (Kawai and Arahama 1958, Kusano 1960, Jwanami *et al.* 1968).

It was believed earlier, that neonatal herpes results from contact with oral herpes of the mother or the nurse, although it was suggested by some authors (Zuelzer and Stulberg 1952, Colebatch 1956) that it could occur during delivery through the infected birth canal. However, with the recognition of type 2 HVH, concepts regarding etiology, therapy and prophylaxis of the disease have changed.

II Incidence

Until recently, most reported cases of neonatal herpes were diagnosed only at postmortem examination. Now, however, various clinical forms of the disease are recognized and described with increasing frequency.

In their extensive monograph on neonatal herpes, Nahmias *et al.* (1970a) record 156 published cases. According to the estimate, the incidence of the infection ranges from a minimum of 1 in 30 000 to a maximum of 1 in 3 500 deliveries. This estimate is based on data derived from two hospitals for low income patients. Although it is conceivable that the frequency of clinically apparent cases would not be higher elsewhere in the world than that calculated by Nahmias, it is nevertheless probable that the incidence of neonatal herpes varies in different countries and in different populations.

Surveys conducted in the United States indicate that genital herpes is about three times as frequent in pregnant women as in the general adult female population. The incidence of type 2 HVH infection during pregnancy was estimated to vary from 1 in 1500 to 1 in 1000, and even higher in lower socioeconomic groups (Ng *et al.* 1970b; Nahmias *et al.* 1971a; Poste *et al.* 1972).

III Source and route of infection

Neonatal herpes can be divided epidemiologically into three main varieties — prenatal, natal and postnatal. There seems to be no doubt that prenatal infection is caused by herpes, whether genital or nongenital, in the mother. The virus may be transmitted to the fetus either across the placenta or by an ascending route. If neonatal herpes occurs within the first 48 hours after birth the infection was most probably acquired in utero.

At birth, infection of the newborn with herpesvirus usually occurs during delivery through the infected genital tract of the mother. Indeed, the available information suggests that this is the most common mode of transmission of the virus to the infant. Nahmias et al. (1969a, c) present evidence indicating that type 2 HVH is responsible for 90 percent of cases of neonatal herpes. Furthermore, it is known that 95 percent of cases of genital herpes are caused by the same type of virus. This clearly indicates a close link between genital herpes of the mother and neonatal infection (Hudson and McFarland 1969).

Postnatally, the infant may be infected by the mother but also by other persons. In such cases genital herpes may not be the principal etiologic agent. It is quite probable that most cases of postnatal herpes are caused by nongenital infections involving the mouth (Quilligan and Wilson 1951; Bird et al. 1962, 1963; Neiman et al. 1964; Jack and Perry 1959) and skin (McDougal et al. 1954). However, since most cases of postnatal herpes were described before the two types of HVH were recognized it seems reasonable to assume that type 1 HVH may be the predominant cause of postnatal infection. Nonetheless, further studies are needed to clarify this point.

The possibility of nosocomial spread of herpesvirus type 2 from one infant to another within a hospital nursery, although uncommon, may constitute an added risk to the newborn infant if nursery techniques among infants are compromised (Francis et al. 1975). Herpes virus type 2 encephalitis in two neonates born within one month of mothers who lived in the same household was recently described in Canada (Allen et al. 1976).

There is little doubt that *herpetic infection of the mother is the principal source of the virus for the infant.* The possible routes of virus transmission have been diagrammed by Nahmias et al. (1970a). This is shown in Fig. 11. The mother as a source of infection is excluded only in cases in which antibodies to HVH cannot be detected in maternal serum several weeks after delivery.

An analysis of the 176 cases presented by Nahmias et al. (1971a,c) indicates that the source of infection was unknown in 57 percent of patients whereas in the remaining 43 percent evidence of maternal herpes was obtained.

In the latter group, 69 percent of cases of neonatal herpes were due to genital infection of the mother and only 13 percent to nongenital infection of the mother. In 12 percent of cases the site of maternal herpetic infection was unknown, in the remaining 6 the source of the virus was not the mother (Fig. 11).

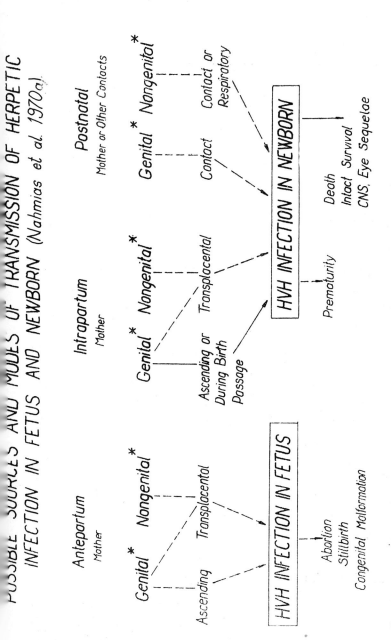

POSSIBLE SOURCES AND MODES OF TRANSMISSION OF HERPETIC INFECTION IN FETUS AND NEWBORN (Nahmias et al. 1970a)

Fig. 11. Possible sources and modes of transmission of herpetic infection in fetus and newborn (Nahmias *et al.* 1970a).

* Clinical or Subclinical (either primary or recurrent)   ———▶ Substantial Evidence   – – – ▶ Suggestive Evidence

Failure to recognize the source of infection is probably due to the fact that many maternal infections are asymptomatic and that the cervix may be involved in the absence of lesions of the external genitalia.

The ascending route of infection is possible in cases of ruptured membranes.

From a number of studies it appears that maternally derived antibodies to HVH do not protect the newborn from infection. There is evidence indicating that some newborns die of herpetic infection in spite of the presence of passively acquired antibodies to either type 1 or type 2 virus or both (Nahmias *et al.* 1969c). There are many problems yet to be solved. For example, virtually no information exists on the number of neonates who are unequivocally exposed to the virus but do not develop the clinical disease. The development of infection may depend on the amount of virus presented to the fetus or newborn. Apparently, a critical level of virus is needed to establish infection. This may be the reason why some newborns do not develop clinical disease even though they were in direct contact with the infected genital tract (Yen *et al.* 1965, Stein and Siciliano 1966, Gagnon 1968, Nahmias *et al.* 1971a).

From the reported cases it appears evident that neonatal herpes may occur as a result of recurrent as well as primary infection of the mother. However, there are observations suggesting that the newborns most at risk are those whose mothers contract primary infection, when the infection lasts longer and the lesions are more extensive then in recurrent lesions. In addition, the risk of abortion and premature delivery is higher in the presence of primary infection (Nahmias *et al.* 1970a). The time of the occurrence of herpetic infection during pregnancy is another important factor. When herpetic infection occurs after 32 weeks of pregnancy the risk for the infant is no less than 10 percent (Nahmias *et al.* 1971a). Maximal risk occurs when genital herpes is present at the time of delivery. Under these circumstances a risk of 80 percent is reported in the literature, based on retrospective surveys, but in a prospective survey Nahmias *et al.* (1971a) found the minimum risk to be 42 percent.

IV Incubation

It was not long ago that the incubation period of neonatal herpes represented an enigma (Langvad and Voigt 1963). In primary herpetic infection of the oral cavity resulting most probably from type 1 HVH, the incubation period was found to vary from 2 to 12 days, with a mean of 6.2±2.7 days (Juretić 1960, 1966). From the published data covering more than 160 cases of neonatal herpetic infection, most of which were contracted during passage through the birth canal, the incubation period of neonatal herpes should not be difficult to calculate. Nevertheless, only scant information is available on this subject. However, most workers agree that clinical disease occurs between the third and the seventh postnatal day (Langvad and Voigt 1963, Overall and Glasgow 1970, Poste et al. 1972). Nahmias et al. (1970a) consider a period of 6 days as the most common. From an analysis of 85 published cases, Sorice (1971) concludes that clinical disease occurred within the first 3 to 10 days of postnatal life in 75 percent; in 14 percent of the patients the disease developed within the first 48 hours after birth, suggesting a prenatal infection. However, in 11 percent of patients in whom disease developed after the first 10 days of life, postnatal infection was most probable.

Data on the incubation period as summarized from the available information on 53 cases are presented in Fig. 12. It can be seen that the incubation period varies from 2 to 11 days with a mean of 5.8±1.9 days.

Comparison between the data presented in Fig. 12. and those obtained from a larger series of patients with primary oral herpetic infection (Table 1) shows that the patterns and mean incubation periods are very similar.

Table 1. *Comparison between incubation periods in days of primary oral infection in children and neonatal herpes*

Infection	Number of cases	Mean incubation period	Standard deviation	Range
Primary oral infection	139	6.1	±2.6	2—12
Neonatal herpes	53	5.8	±1.9	2—12

V Clinical features

Neonatal herpes is characterized by a fulminant and septic course. Because of the very high fatality rate, Debré et al. (1955) called the disease *"lethal herpes."*

5

66

Until recently, most reported cases of neonatal herpes were diagnosed at post-mortem examination and were described as generalized or disseminated forms of HVH infection with or with-

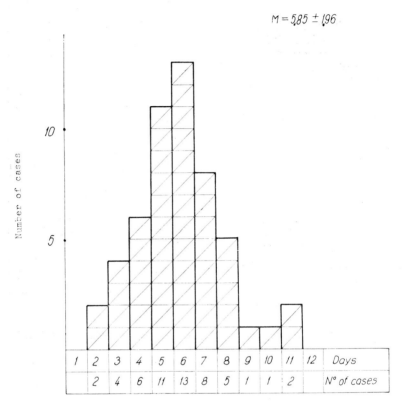

$M = 5,85 \pm 1,96$

Fig. 12. Incubation period of neonatal herpes as resulting from 53 cases reported in the literature.

out involvement of the central nervous system (Nahmias 1972). During the past few years, however, localized forms of herpetic infection involving tissues originating from the ectoderm (CNS, eyes, skin and mucous membranes) have been recognized with increasing frequency. On the other hand, asymptomatic forms of neonatal herpes have been encountered only rarely (Künzer *et al.* 1966; Sanders and Cramblett 1968) and there is no information regarding their frequency (Gerola 1972). Without entering into details of these considerations, we may sum up (Table 2) the various forms of neonatal herpes as classified by Nahmias *et al.* (1970) (Table 2).

Table 2. *Clinical features of neonatal herpes* (Bassed on the classification of Nahmias *et al.* 1970a).

Clinical form	Host-virus relation	Prognosis
I. Generalized or disseminated forms (polyvisceritis)	Involvement of most organs	Very poor; exeptions very rare
II. Localized forms 1. CNS 2. Eyes 3. Skin 4. Mucous membranes 5. Combined	Only tissues originating from the ectoderm are involved	Poor if CNS involved. Otherwise better with possible sequelae
III. Asymptomatic forms	Absence of clinical signs	Good but follow up required

Generalized or disseminated forms usually begin a few days after birth. The onset of the disease is usually accompained by non-specific constitutional signs including anorexia, vomiting, diarrhea, hypoactivity and temperature alterations (hypo-and hyperpyrexia). According to Miller *et al.* (1970) the principal specific symptoms indicating a disseminated form of neonatal herpes are respiratory difficulties, hepatomegaly with or without jaundice, splenomegaly, hemorrhagic diathesis, vesicular skin lesions, symptoms originating from CNS involvement, and ocular and oral cavity lesions. Post-mortal examination confirms that the disseminated form of herpes infection affects primarily the liver in almost every patient. Clinically, however, hepatomegaly and jaundice have been recognized in only one-third of the reported cases. The central nervous system was involved in 25—45 percent of the patients. Involvement of the CNS was most commonly recognized by convulsions, bulging fontanelle, opisthotonus, alterations of muscle tone and coma. Evidently, lumbar puncture is always indicated when the disseminated form of the disease is suspected even though there are no clinical signs of CNS involvement. In the presence of CNS involvement the virus can often be recovered from the spinal fluid, and pleocytosis, frequently associated with elevated protein levels, is regularly observed. Electroencephalograms done in some cases showed typical periods of hypo- and hyperactivity (Pettay *et al.* 1972). However, the specificity of EEG findings has been questioned by some workers.

The findings most helpful in the diagnosis of neonatal herpes include the presence of scalp vesicles (Echeverria *et al.* 1973), keratoconjunctivitis (Berkovich and Ressel 1966) and ulcerations in the oral cavity. Ulcerations of the esophagus have often been diagnosed, but only at autopsy (Langvad and Voigt 1963, Wright and Miller 1965, Laboureau et al. 1973).

Hemorrhagic diathesis was documented in one third of the published cases. Earlier it was believed that bleeding resulted from septicemia and damage to the liver. Recently, however, evidence has been obtained suggesting that hemorrhagic diathesis results from *disseminated intravascular coagulation — DIC* (Gagnon 1968, Hathaway et al. 1969, Robinson and Kauffman 1969, Shershow et al. 1969, Miller et al. 1970). The process of consumptive coagulopathy in cases of neonatal herpes has been documented by thrombocytopenia, fibrinogenopenia, reduced levels of factors V and VIII, hypoprothrombinemia, prolonged thromboplastin and thrombin times, prolonged bleeding time and the presence of fibrin degradation products. All this suggests that herpesvirus belongs to the group of agents that can provoke DIC in the neonate.

Heyne (1974) draws attention to the possible role of the observed phagocytic dysfunction of granulocytes (necrobiotic cells) in the pathogenesis of generalized HVH infection, especially in the triggering of disseminated intravascular coagulation and in the occasional combination with microbiologic superinfection.

Thus far, only four survivors of disseminated herpes infection have been reported. Two of them had no apparent sequelae, whereas of the remaining two, one survived with hypoadrenalism and severe CNS and ocular damage (Bahrami et al. 1966) and the other with neurologic sequelae (Golden et al. 1969).

The absence of visceral involvement is typical of *localized forms of neonatal herpes infection*. Up to the present time, about 50 cases of localized forms of the disease have been described. *Involvement of the central nervous system*, which represents the most severe form, was diagnosed in about one-half of the cases. The onset of the disease is characterized by convulsions. In cerebrospinal fluid, pleocytosis is the rule and protein levels are usually elevated. Electroencephalogram records in a few cases show abnormalities (Epstein and Crouch 1954, Lamy et al. 1960). Generally, the presence of CNS involvement augurs a poor prognosis. The affected patients either died (44 percent) or survived with severe sequelae including microcephaly, hydrocephaly, porencephaly and psychomotor retardation. However, one survivor with involvement of the CNS but without apparent clinical or pathologic sequelae has also been reported (Gershon et al. 1972).

The *eyes* may be the only site of herpetic infection in the infant. They may, however, be affected in association with herpetic encephalitis (Florman and Mindlin 1952, Berkovich and Ressel 1966). Herpetic ocular lesions in the neonate usually begin with keratoconjunctivitis and keratitis (Bobo *et al.* 1970). Chorioretinitis may develop alone and become apparent after several months (Proto and Tedesco 1966, Hagler *et al.* 1969, Nahmias and Hagler 1972).

The most frequently encountered form of neonatal herpes is that of vesicular *skin lesions* (Torphy *et al.* 1970, Frangini and Matucci 1971). When these are confined to the skin, the prognosis is usually good. However, such patients require careful follow-up because vesicular skin lesions in the newborn may be associated with infection of the eyes or CNS or both that is clinically ina-parent at that time (Nahmias *et al.* 1969c). Vesicular skin lesions have been observed to recur repeatedly for several years after birth (Nahmias *et al.* 1970a).

Oral herpes in the neonate usually results from postnatal herpetic infection.

VI Prevention

The first step in preventing neonatal herpes is to avoid genital infection of the mother during the last trimester of pregnancy. In connection with this it is important that males with penile le-sions abstain from having sexual relations with pregnant women (Zavorall *et al.* 1970).

Next, any unexplained pyrexia during pregnancy should be investigated because of the possibility that it may be caused by herpesvirus infection. Further, periodic examinations of the genital tract and virus cultures from any ulcerative or vesicular lesions should be made in pregnant women (MacCallum 1959). If maternal genital herpes is present near term, local application of antiviral drugs such as 5-iodo-2-oxyuridine (IDU) may be tried even though the efficacy of topical therapy has not been unequivocally demon-strated (Nahmias and Roizman 1973). The use of gama globulin has been advocated as a preventive measure for infants undoubt-edly exposed to herpesvirus. However, in spite of gamma glob-ulin therapy, disseminated neonatal herpesvirus infection ensued in the great majority of cases (Zuelzer and Stulberg 1952, Wheeler and Huffiness 1965). Similar attempts at preventing herpetic sto-matitis in children and experimental ocular infection in rabbits also failed to produce conclusive evidence regarding the efficacy of gamma globulin (Juretić and Ribarić 1970). It has been suggest-ed that better results might be obtained by the use of a hyperim-mune type 2 gamma globulin if it were available. At present, pooled gamma globulin in large doses (20—40 ml) is being used for the mother because of the theoretical possibility that it might prevent blood-borne herpesvirus infection in the nonimmune infant (Nahmias *et al.* 1971a).

Evidently, the most successful way to prevent postnatal infection is to keep the newborn away from the source of HVH. Therefore it is important that persons with herpetic lesions avoid contact with the newborn infant. In mothers with genital herpes present at a time near term, delivery by Cesarean section has been recommended as one of the most efficient measures to prevent neonatal herpes. However, even this approach may be unsuccessful in protecting the newborn if the membranes have ruptured, because of the increased opportunity for an ascending infection. Therefore, it is often advisable to perform the operation before the membrane rupture or at the latest within the first 6 hours after rupture (Poste *et al.* 1972; Amstey, 1970). Recently, Nahmias and Roizman (1973) reported results on the efficacy of Cesarean section in protecting the neonate from HVH infection. Of the 16 reported cases only one was unsuccessful.

Amniocentesis and amniotic fluid culture may provide an important clue to early diagnosis of intrauterine herpesvirus infection. If HVH is detected in the amniotic fluid the efficacy of abdominal delivery may be doubtful. On the basis of the results of viral cultures Amstey (1970) proposes guidelines for the management of problematic cases (Fig. 13).

The history of genital herpes during pregnancy and particularly around the time of delivery is also important in the diagnosis of neonatal herpes. It is interesting that some cases of neonatal herpes were diagnosed on the basis of maternal infection even before the disease was clinically manifested (Wheeler and Huffiness 1965, Hutfield 1966a).

Detection of herpesvirus antigen in cervical smears by immunofluorescent antibodies is undoubtedly a valuable guide to diagnosis in suspected cases (Pettay *et al.* 1972).

The appearance of vesicles in the oral cavity or on the scalp of the newborn is often decisive for the prompt recognition of herpetic infection. In addition, it supports the view that the infection is most commonly acquired during the passage through the infected birth canal. Indeed, the head and the mouth of the infant usually have the longest period of contact with the infected cervix (Echeverria *et al.* 1973).

Herpesvirus type 2 has been isolated with increasing frequency, not only from the skin lesions, eyes and mucous membranes of infected newborns but also from the blood, urine, and cerebrospinal fluid (Chang *et al.* 1966). At autopsy, the virus can be recovered from almost every organ. The lesions all show the characteristic histologic picture of intranuclear inclusion bodies and focal necrosis. Necrotic foci are most prominent in the liver, brain, adrenals and kidneys. In recent years, histologic analysis has been greatly facilitated by the use of electron microscopy and fluorescent antibody techniques (Torphy *et al.* 1970, Nahmias *et al.* 1970a). Indirect immunofluorescence and radioimmunological methods have been developed recently to detect HSV antibodies in the IgM, IgG and IgA classes of immunoglobulins.

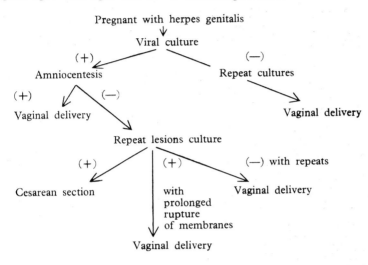

Fig. 13. Summary of the management of patients with genital herpes infection in pregnancy based on positive (+) and negative (—) viral cultures (Amstey 1970).

Detection of specific herpesvirus antibodies is more important epidemiologically than as an aid in the diagnosis of neonatal herpes. It may take repeated serologic examinations over a period of several months to reveal a relation between antibodies passively acquired from the mother and those produced by the infant. However, since antibodies of the IgM variety are not normally transmitted across the placenta the finding of specific IgM antibodies shortly after birth may be taken as indicative of neonatal herpes infection. Thus IgM HSV antibodies can be employed to provide evidence of a clinically undiagnosed HSV-2 perinataly acquired infection. Such IgM antibodies appear within 1—4 wk. after birth and persist for at least 6 months (Nahmias and Josey, 1976).

VII Therapy

The high mortality rate and high percentage of severe neurologic sequelae that result from disseminated neonatal herpes justify therapeutic attempts with antiviral agents even though they may be toxic.

The agent that is most frequently used is *5-iodo-2-deoxy-uridine* (IDU). The results of IDU treatment of disseminated neonatal herpes are summarized in Table 3 (Partridge and Millis 1968, MacCallum and Patridge 1968; Tuffli and Nahmias, 1969). Apparently, such therapy does not do much to interfere with the course of the disease. But it should be noted that it was initiated too late in most cases. The drug was administered intravenously for 5 to 7 days at a daily dose of 50 to 100 mg per kilogram of body weight. Although toxic effects of the drug were not readily apparent, a mild depression of myelopoesis was nevertheless observed (Golden *et al.* 1969). Generally, the results of IDU-treatment are hard to evaluate because of the fatal outcome in most cases. Besides, the therapy was instituted at various times after the onset of the disease (Gershon *et al.* 1972). Antiviral therapy appears to be efficient only in patients in whom the diagnosis is established early, before irreversible brain damage occurs (Charnock and Cramblett 1970). However, the problem of the therapeutic efficacy of IDU treatment in type 2 HVH infections still remains unclear. Several in vitro studies have demonstrated that type 2 HVH is more resistant to IDU treatment than type 1 (Nahmias and Dowdle 1968).

Table 3. *Results of IDU treatment of patients with severe forms of neonatal herpes treated*

	Number of cases	Fatal outcome	Alive with severe	Sequelae mild	Authors
Disseminated					Patridge and Millis
	2		2		1968
					Golden *et al.* 1969
Localized					Tuffli and Nahmias, 1969
	6	2	2+	2	
					Pettay *et al.* 1972
Total	8	2	4	2	

+ One of the patients subsequently died of bacterial infection.

Another agent with potential antiviral activity is *polyinosinic-cydilic acid (Poly-IC)*, a double stranded RNA that has been shown to stimulate interferon production. The preparation was applied, with at least some success, to a 5-months old infant with generalized herpetic infection (Catalano 1969, Catalano and Baron 1970).

The recent development of *interferon* inducers as prophylatic and therapeutic antiherpesvirus drugs suggests another possible mode of therapy in this disease. The combination of passive antibody administration (hyperimmune type 1 or 2 HVH antiserum) and either IDU or interferon stimulation might be of greater therapeutic benefit in disseminated herpes neonatorum (Catalano *et al.* 1971).

There are reports of three patients with HVH-2 and one with HVH-1 with neonatal infection of the central nervous system who were not given antiviral drugs and who did not develop brain damage (Gershon *et al*, 1972, Torphy *et al.* 1970, Frenz *et al.* 1974).

It is obvious, however, that controlled studies are required in order to evaluate the therapeutic efficacy of these and other antiviral drugs in HVH infection of the newborn (Tuflli and Nahmias 1969, Gershon *et al.* 1972).

It is also quite apparent that in addition to antiviral drugs several other therapeutic measures should be used. First, hypoglycemia and alterations of the acid-base balance need correction with the appropriate intravenous fluids. Second, adrenal insufficiency which is typical of disseminated herpes infection should be diagnosed early and treated adequately (Bahrani *et al.* 1966). In patients with disseminated herpes infection associated with intravenous coagulation, heparin therapy and replacement of coagulation factors are indicated (Miller *et al.* 1970, Shershow *et al.* 1969). In addition, appropiate antibiotics must be given in order to combat secondary bacterial infection.

In a recent study published by Ch'ien *et al.* (1975), 13 neonates with HVH infection were treated with parenteral administration of *adenine arabinoside (ara-A)*. Eight infants (4 with disseminated and 4 with localized skin disease) with skin vesicles as the earliest sign of infection received ara-A early on, within 3 days of the onset of neurologic signs. All survived with no neurologic deficit at 6 months to 1 year of age. There was no apparent toxicity of ara-A to the bone marrow, liver or kidney. In order to evaluate the true effect of ara-A on the natural course of neonatal herpes infection, a sufficient number of patients must be studied. A large scale multi-institutional study with double-blind protocol is now in progress (JAMA 1974, Ch'ien *et al.* 1975).

Chapter 6

DISSEMINATED HERPES SIMPLEX INFECTION OF INFANTS AND OLDER CHILDREN

Zuelzer and Stulberg (1952) were the first to describe wide-spread herpetic lesions in the viscera of three older infants. Focal necrotic lesions were invariably found in the liver. Typical herpetic stomatitis preceded herpetic lesions. The authors recorded viremia as a regular phenomenon in primary herpetic gingivostomatitis of infants. Necrotic adrenal lesions have been noted in association with eczema herpeticum (Pugh *et al.* 1954, 1955; Brain *et al.* 1957). Hepatoadrenal necrosis was the prominent feature in both disseminated forms of herpetic disease (neonatal and in infants).

Eight cases of disseminated herpes simplex virus infection in children have been reported from Cape Town (McKenzie *et al.* 1959). The report was based on the autopsy findings and histologic examination of 8 patients aged 9—16 months, in 3 of whom the diagnosis was confirmed by isolation of the virus from the tissues. In addition to stomatitis, they all showed similar lesions in the adrenals consisting of multiple necrotic foci around which cells containing characteristic intranuclear inclusion bodies could be found. In 7 cases there was severe malnutrition.

Hansen (1961) and McKenzie (1961) made independent retrospective studies of 121 cases of herpetic disease treated in two hospitals in South Africa. Thirty three of the patients died and in 16 of them (including the 8 previously cited cases) generalized herpes simplex infection was found at autopsy. The high incidence of infection in the lower socioeconomic groups (all patients were negro or other colored children) is pointed out. The age range in this series was from 2 to 36 months.

In a further study involving another 16 patients from South Africa, widespread distribution of the virus has been demonstrated. The concentration of the virus was found to vary greatly in different tissues and from patient to patient (Becker *et al.* 1963). All but one of the 16 patients were thought to have encephalitis on clinical

examination. Fatal infantile generalized herpes differs from neonatal generalized herpes, the former being associated almost
invariably with severe malnutrition (Fig. 14).

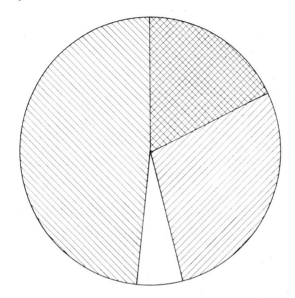

		Number	Percent
	Kwashiorkor	46	49
	Severe Malnutrition	17	18
	Underweight	25	27
	Well Nourished	6	6

Fig. 14. The association of fatal postneonatal herpetic dissemination and
severe malnutrition in 93 cases from South Africa (Kipps *et al.* 1967)

A correlation between the socioeconomic status of the population and the incidence of herpetic antibodies was confirmed by
a comparative study by Becker (1966) carried out in Cape Town
on individuals belonging to three racial groups.

Tucker and Scofield (1961) report an isolated case of fatal
herpetic infection in a child who had developed measles 3 weeks
earlier. The importance of the measles as a determinant of the out-

come of primary herpesvirus infections in children has been stressed by Armengaud *et al.* (1963) and by Kipps *et al.* (1967). In the study by Kipps 17 percent of all fatal cases occurred after measles while in the study of Armengaud all 13 (100 percent) fatal cases occurred after an attack of measles.

A generalized fatal herpetic infection in a 9-month old infant after measles and enterocolitis has been reported from Yugoslavia (Beloševic and Hirtzler 1968).

Especially frequent and dangerous is the combination of the two predisposing factors: malnutrition and a post-measles state. Other acute infections such as whooping cough may also precede herpetic infection and possibly predispose to the fatal outcome.

Reviewing 33 cases of disseminated herpesvirus infection (in infants and children up to 34 months of age), Becker *et al.* (1968) discuss the pathogenesis of the disease, and describe three phases. In the first phase small amounts of the virus produce primary lesions, usually in the mouth, which result in minimal viremia. In the second phase typical herpetic lesions develop in the viscera (most often in the liver and adrenals). In the third phase the lesions progress and a feedback of virus into the blood stream produces a second and more massive viremia. Most deaths in the series reported by them occurred during the florid stage of the disease.

The causes and mechanism of death in disseminated herpes may be different. In some cases hypoglycemia was the main cause of the fatal outcome (Becker *et al.* 1968).

All cited surveys of the incidence of disseminated herpes infection have been concerned with type 1 HVH, so that very little information is as yet available regarding the incidence of type 2 strains, especially in Africa. On that continent neonatal herpetic infection resulting from infection with type 2 is extremely rare; only two cases have been described (Kipps *et al.* 1967; Templeton 1970). There are two possible explanations for this: either all mothers are immune or the causative virus is very rare.

In Uganda, Templeton (1970) recorded five cases of disseminated herpes in malnourished children.

The reason for the apparently higher incidence of fatal disseminated herpes infections in South Africa is almost certainly that HVH is a much more common disease in underdeveloped regions than is at present recognized. The retrospective histopathologic study of Rose and Becker (1972) has shown that disseminated HVH infections in the neonatal form and in association with malnution in older children occurred in South Africa before 1957. Only a greater awareness of this disease and the use of different diagnostic approaches, histologic and virologic, will lead to a better knowledge of its true incidence.

At autopsy the most common lesions were found in the liver, adrenals and esophagus; this is shown by the data in Table 1.

Table 1. *Involvement of organs in 48 cases of disseminated postneonatal herpes infections* (Sorice 1971)

Organ	No of cases	Percentage
Liver	40	83.3
Adrenal	33	68.7
Lungs	7	14.5
CNS	3	6.2
Esophagus	31	64.4
Kidneys	1	2.0
Spleen	3	6.2
Heart	1	2.1
Gastrointestinal tract (bowels, stomach)	4	8.3
Larynx and trachea	2	4.2

An analysis of clinical symptoms in the 51 cases published in the medical literature shows that the disease is most often characterized by hyperpyrexia, hepatomegaly and stomatitis, as shown in Table 2.

Table 2. *Clinical symptoms in 51 cases of disseminated postneonatal herpes infections* (Sorice 1971)

Symptom	No of cases	Percent
Fever	51	100
Hepatomegaly	41	80.4
Stomatitis	40	78.4
Respiratory failure	17	33.3
Hemorrhagic diathesis	22	43.1
Herpes of the skin	12	23.5
Neurological symptoms	11	21.6
Jaundice, splenomegaly diarrhea etc.	12	23.5

The virus was isolated from various organs, most often from the liver and adrenals, but also from the lungs, CNS, spleen, kidneys, heart, pharynx and blood.

The fatality rate among the published cases of disseminated non-neonatal herpes infections was as high as that in neonatal herpes. Up to now only two cases without a fatal ending have been described (Sorice 1971). The disease develops very fast and death occurred in 85 percent of cases within 10 days. In most of the cases the diagnosis was made after death.

The prognosis is especially bad perhaps because the infection often occurs in association with prematurity and malnutrition, with other infectious diseases such as measles and whooping cough (diseases that weaken the body's resistance), with congenital or acquired immunodeficiency, such as the Wiscott-Aldrich syndrome or Hodgkin's disease, with immunosuppressive therapy, or with extensive skin alteration resulting from eczema or burns.

Esophagitis herpetica was first published by Fingerland *et al.* (1952) in autopsy findings in five adults without malignancies. Until recently the *involvement of the lower respiratory tract* with herpesvirus was regarded as extremely rare. The first case was reported by Morgan and Finland in 1949: HVH was isolated from the pulmonary tissue of a patient with atypical pneumonia and erythema exudativum multiforme, but without adequate histologic documentation. Six cases of herpetic involvement of the trachea, bronchi and alveoli have been found in autopsy material selected from 3 000 cases (Herout *et al.* 1966). In a 13-month old girl the virus was isolated from the lung tissue. The child had probable simultaneous infection with morbilli. Concomitant herpetic lesions in the oral cavity or esophagus were present in almost all cases. The possibility of subsequent aspiration has been suggested. Herpetic pneumonia in alcoholic hepatitis treated with corticosteroids has been reported by Caldwell and Porter (1971).

Disseminated herpetic lesions of the respiratory tract and other visceral organs in malignancies, burns and other conditions are dealt with in Chapters 7, 8 and 12.

There are certain common denominators among these groups of susceptible persons: underlying skin disorders, low serum protein levels and a deficient cellular immune responsiveness (Nahmias 1970).

Chapter 7

THE IMMUNOLOGICALLY COMPROMISED HOST

Certain conditions or drugs that compromise immunity competence, particularly cellular immunity, may be associated with increased susceptibility to HVH infection. Notorious examples of this association are predisposing conditions such as eczema, severe malnutrition and measles.

It has long been known that *steroids*, particularly in high and prolonged dosage, can increase the incidence and severity of infections due to bacteria, fungi and viruses. There are several articles describing how steroids unfavorably bias the course of experimental herpesvirus infection in animals (McCoy and Leopold 1960). Sometimes patients with primary systemic amyloidosis (Stroud 1961) or with pemphigus foliaceus (Indgin and Connor 1970) may develop generalized recurrent herpesvirus infection as a result of prednisone therapy. Herpetic pneumonia associated with primary hepatic disease under corticosteroid therapy has been reported (Caldwell and Porter 1971).

St. Geme *et al.* (1965) report an alarming progression of primary herpetic gingivostomatitis in three boys with the familial syndrome of eczema, thrombocytopenia and recurrent infection — the *Wiscott-Aldrich syndrome*. Serologic investigation revealed a very limited and delayed antibody response in all three. Deficient cellular resistance allowed the virus to persist in the tissues of these patients with the induction of partial to complete immunologic tolerance. Evans and Holzel (1970) describe three attacks of disseminated herpes in a girl with eczema and low serum IgM (a possible female variant of the Wiscott-Aldrich syndrome).

An association between *herpes simplex and malignancy* has been suggested by Berg and Wyburn-Mason. Berg (1955) described 12 cases of fatal esophageal herpes in cancer patients. Wyburn-Mason (1957) reported a series of cases of carcinoma of the lip preceded by herpes simplex. Berg's observations are confirmed by a review of 2573 autopsies made in Chicago, where Moses and Cheatham (1963) described herpetic esophagitis in 12 cases. The highest incidence (7 of 227 or 3.1 percent) of cases in which sections of the esophagus were involved was found in patients over the age of 50 with malignancies. Two cases of histologically documented herpetic involvement of the trachea, bronchi and alveoli found in autopsy material associated with a malignant disease have been reported by Czech authors (Herout et al. 1966).

Bacterial, fungal and viral infections are common complications in patients with *hematologic malignancies*. The impression emerging from clinical experience is that infections due to HVH are more common or severe in patients with lymphoma. The first case of herpesvirus from skin lesions of a patient with myelogenous leukemia was reported by Solomon (1961). However the diagnosis of the malignant disorder in this patient was not made until postmortem.

Casazza et al. (1966) report 8 cases of disseminated HVH infection among 139 patients who died of lymphoma. The diagnosis was made solely on the basis of histopathologic findings. Generalized vesicular exanthem associated with an acute febrile episode due to HVH has been described in four adult patients with hematologic malignancy (Rendtorf and Fowinkle 1969, Lynfield et al. 1969).

Bean and Fusaro (1969) describe a chronic type of cutaneous herpetic ulcer (herpes phagedena) occurring on the face, especially about the lips, nose and eyelids, on the buttocks and on the anogenital area of patients with hematologic malignancies. A very similar case of extensive and atypical skin manifestations of herpesvirus infection in a child with acute leukemia is reported by Nishimura et al. (1972).

Perhaps the most comprehensive study of HVH infections in patients with hematologic malignancies is that published by Muller et al. (1972). They made a comparative analysis of 51 cases (20 at the Mayo Clinic and 31 collected from the literature). Herpesvirus infection was a complication in 12 patients with Hodgkin's disease, in 12 with lymphosarcoma, in 9 with chronic lymphatic leukemia, in 6 with myelogenous leukemia, in 5 with reticulum cell sarcoma, in 2 with acute leukemia, in 2 with unspecified leukemia, in 2 with mycosis fungoides and in 1 with chronic myelofibrosis. In the clinical spectrum of herpetic disease there were 24 localized cutaneous syndromes, 17 disseminated cutaneous eruptions, and 10 visceral disseminations and esophageal lesions. Muller et al. (1972) stress the vulnerability of patients with hematologic malignancies to the development of HVH infections affecting the skin and mucous membranes. They suggest that disease-related immunologic impairment and massive suppression of immunologic defense mechanisms by chemotherapy are major associated factors.

Infections due to HVH after kidney *transplantation* have been reported on several occasions. Montgomerie *et al.* (1969) describe a severe HVH infection in 4 patients who died after receiving kidney transplants. In all of these patients typical herpes labialis progressed to involve adjacent areas, face, eye, nostrils, mouth and esophagus; all were also infected with cytomegalovirus. The possibility that these patients had primary herpes simplex infections was excluded by the demonstration that the titer of complement fixing antibodies had not increased significantly during the illness. The immunity deficiency responsible for the extensive development of HVH infection was not identified. It was probably both suppression of humoral antibody production and delayed hypersensitivity resulting from immunosuppressive therapy (with azothioprine and corticosteroids). The association of progressive herpes simplex infection and terminal pneumonitis due to cytomegalovirus and *pneumocystitis carinii* was later described by Crosby *et al.* (1969).

On the other hand Spencer and Anderson (1970) noted that in a group of 83 recipients of renal allograft, herpes simplex lesions appeared to be no more common after transplantation than before in those patients who were subject to recurrent attacks. Pien *et al.* (1973) report 17 kidney transplant recipients with 9 seroconversions for HVH antibodies. No statistical correlation was found between the incidence of renal allograft rejection and the development of viral seroconversions.

Considering the paucity of reports *HVH infection involving the lower respiratory tract*, it is interesting to note the case reported by Douglas *et al.* (1969) of herpes simplex pneumonia occurring in an allotransplanted lung. The etiology was documented by isolation of HVH from the sputum as well as from lung tissue obtained by biopsy and at autopsy. Treatment with cytarabin failed to eradicate the virus or to produce significant clinical improvement.

All the cited reports suggest that impairment of the host's general cellular reactivity by combined immunosuppresive therapy may be a hazard for every transplant patient (St. Geme *et al.* 1965, Montgomerie *et al.* 1969, Crosby *et al.* 1969, Douglas *et al.* 1969).

Merigan and Stevens (1971) have surveyed all viral infections in man associated with aquired immunologic deficiency states. In Table 1 we have attemped to compile all clinical states of immunosuppression associated with herpetic disease.

6

Table 1. *Clinical states of immunosupression associated with HVH disease* (modified after Merigan and Stevens 1971.)

Organ transplantation
Malignancies including
  lymphomas
Drug therapy (cortico-
  steroids and other)
X-irradiation

Other states associated with
immunosuppression (measles,
malnutrition, burns, eczema,
prematurity, splenectomy,
miscellaneous skin diseases
and the like).

Chapter 8

ECZEMA HERPETICUM

In 1887 Kaposi described a generalized vesicular skin eruption occurring as a complication of an infantile eczema for which he first suggested the name "eczema herpetiforme" although he suspected a fungus as the cause. Descriptions of the clinical course of this disease found in the modern literature add little to his vivid description of more than 90 years ago. In 1898, Juliusberg reported what appears to have been the same disease (cit. by Freund 1934) and drew attention to the close resemblance of the individual lesions to vaccination pustules. Since then the disease has been called "pustulosis acute varioliformis" or "pustulosis acuta vacciniformis" or more often the "Kaposi-Juliusberg syndrome". At the time, however a number of bacteria and at least one of the filtrable viruses (vaccinia) were considered as the etiologic agents (Freund 1934). For about 50 years a number of causes were suspected but never proved. Esser (1941) and Seidenberg (1941) contributed the first evidence that the virus of herpes simplex caused Kaposi varicelliform eruption in at least some cases. During the Second World War a number of reports from the United States lent support to a herpetic etiology of the disease. Following the demonstration that the disease could result from infection with herpesvirus it was suggested that the term "Kaposi's varicelliform eruption" should be abandoned in favor of "eczema herpeticum" (Lynch 1945, Lynch and Steves 1947) or herpes simplex complicating eczema. By observing a series of cases Lynch came to the conclusion that herpes virus infection can be superimposed on eczematous skin. In a study of some cases of Kaposi's syndrome Ruchman and Dodd (1948) obtained evidence that this entity is in all probability a manifestation of primary infection with herpesvirus in persons with eczema. Although infantile eczema is a common disease, and the virus of herpes is widely distributed, eczema herpeticum remains a relatively rare condition (Barrow 1954). Some clinicians are of the opinion that eczema vaccinatum and eczema herpeticum can probably be distinguished clinically in the majority of instances. The vesicles of eczema vaccinatum are as a rule fewer, larger and tenser, and more of them are pustular or umbilicated. In addition the eruption and the general illness last longer than in cases of eczema herpeticum (Lynch 1945, Lausecker 1953, 1955).

There are comparatively few accounts of Kaposi's syndrome being transmitted from one patient to another. In 1936 McLaghlan and Gillespie observed an epidemic occurring on a children's skin ward (cit. by Simpson 1953). No attempt was made to isolate a virus but only one of the children had been vaccinated. These authors noted three large pustular bullae on the forearms. Examples of direct transmission of eczema vaccinatum have been repeatedly reported. Esser (1941) was the first to report an outbreak of eczema herpeticum in an infants' ward, where 4 out of 8 children with eczema developed herpetic eruption. From two of them herpesvirus was recovered and identified by Seidenberg (1941). In 1948, Sims and French (cit. by Simpson 1953) reported a small epidemic (probably 6 cases) of eczema herpeticum, and presented laboratory evidence of infection by herpes virus.

The development of sore throat, vesicopustules, and other herpetic lesions in the attending staff has also been reported (Barton and Brunsting 1944, cit. by Barrow 1954; Simpson 1953). Pugh et al. (1955) report the occurrence of herpetic infection in four children treated for eczema. In the same ward two of the nurses became infected. Two cases of ward infection from eczema herpeticum have been recorded by Puretić (cit. by Juretić 1970).

As in other forms of disease caused by herpesvirus, eczema herpeticum may occur as either a primary or a recurrent disease (Wheeler et al. 1966). The primary infection is stated to be more severe, with a higher mortality rate. However, it is often impossible to distinguish between primary and recurrent infection on purely clinical grounds. Serologic studies are necessary for differentiation between the two forms.

Primary eczema herpeticum would be expected to be a serious disease with viremia and frequent involvement of internal organs. In Kaposi's original description one of the six patients had an overt neurologic disease (Kaposi 1893). One patient in a series presented by Wenner (1944) had involuntary movements and seizures. Pugh et al. (1955) observed typical herpetic lesions in a fatal case of eczema herpeticum in an 11-month-old infant with evidence of hematogenous dissemination of the virus to the liver and adrenals, in conjunction with atypical pulmonary necrosis. Monif et al. (1968) found visceral infection by HVH and probable CNS involvement in a 5-month-old infant with eczema herpeticum who died of an intercurrent Pseudomonas septicemia. Bacterial involvement of the skin and internal organs together with extensive cutaneous malfunction from the widespread inflammation sometimes has a bad prognosis, particularly if the patients are receiving corticosteroid treatment (Jank and Söltz-Szötz 1966; Söltz-Szötz and Fanta 1974).

The prognosis of eczema herpeticum depends upon the virulence of the virus, the susceptibility of the host, the nature and extent of previous skin trauma and secondary infection with its ensuing complications. The mortality rate is variable, ranging from 10 to 20 percent. The prognosis in adults is better (Söltz-Szötz 1963, Graciansky *et al.* 1970).

The Kaposi syndrome caused by HVH has been described in a number of other skin diseases. Doeglas and Moolhuysen (1969) review 6 cases of *Darier's disease* complicated by possible or proven secondary herpes simplex virus infection. In 2 cases primary infection was proved; in the other 4 there was evidence of recurrent infection. Sunburn is reported as a precipitating factor in this condition (Weiss *et al.* 1965).

Since primary infection with herpes simplex is uncommon in adults and the manifestations may mimic various other disorders, its presence as a complication may be overlooked (Fisher and Kibrick 1963, Hitselberg and Burns 1968, Graciansky *et al.* 1970).

The virus isolated from cases of Darier's disease complicated with Kaposi syndrome, has been recognized as being type 1 HVH (Izumi and Goldschmidt 1970).

St. Geme *et al.* (1965) describe disseminated herpetic infection in the Wiscott-Aldrich syndrome. There are reports indicating that generalized cutaneous herpesvirus infection may develop in patients with pemphigus vulgaris and pemphigus foliacecus treated with corticosteroids (Marton and Angyal 1963, cit. by Silverstein and Burnett 1967; Indgin and Connor 1970).

Considering the diversity of skin diseases that may be complicated by HVH or vaccinia infection, Doeglas and Moolhuysen (1969) have suggested that the term "Kaposi's varicelliform eruption" be followed by the name of the underlying skin disease and the name of the causative virus.

Chapter 9

HERPETIC INFECTION OF THE CENTRAL NERVOUS SYSTEM

M. GAZDIK and M. JURETIĆ

Herpesvirus hominis has been implicated as the etiologic agent in a wide varety of central nervous system diseases. The commonest manifestations of CNS infection with herpesvirus in adults are meningitis and encephalitis. Herpetic meningitis is a rather benign disease associated with type 2 HVH. Herpetic encephalitis is a severe, rapidly progressing and often fatal disease associated predominantly with type 1 HVH (Drachman and Adams 1962; Olson *et al.* 1967; Haynes *et al.* 1968; Skoldenberg 1972). In newborn and infants, CNS infection usually occurs in association with systemic involvement (Zuelzer and Stulberg 1952). The possible role of herpesvirus in the etiology of some chronic neurologic diseases such as subacute sclerosing panencephalitis (Dodge and Cure 1956; Kurtzke 1956; Sherman *et al.* 1961), multiple sclerosis (Gudnadottir *et al.* 1964; Dowdle *et al.* 1967), amiotrophic lateral sclerosis (Plummer 1967) and some psychopathic diseases (Cleoburry and Skinner 1971) has also been suggested although never well established (Millar *et al.* 1972).

I. Herpetic meningitis

At the beginning of this century, French workers observed meningeal symptoms in patients with genital or skin infection due to herpesvirus. Nicolau and Poincloux (1924) induced herpetic meningitis in man by intrathecal inoculation of the infectious material. Janbon *et al.* (1942), Armstrong (1943), Afzelius-Alm (1951), and Stadler *et al.* (1973) have reported the isolation of HVH from the cerebrospinal fluid of patients with meningitis.

Most workers hold that herpetic meningitis is not as common as herpetic encephalitis. Afzelius-Alm (1951) states that herpesvirus is responsible for about 20 percent of aseptic meningitis. Other authors give incidences ranging from 0 to 5 percent (Meyer et al. 1970).

Herpetic meningitis is a sporadic disease occurring in both sexes of all ages and in most communities without seasonal variations. It may occur as an isolated disease (Armstrong 1943; Leider et al. 1965), although it has commonly been described in patients with genital herpes (Ravaut and Darre 1904; Afzelius-Alm 1951; Hunt and Comer 1955; Gillot et al. 1958; Duxbury and Lawrence 1959; Terni et al. 1971; Cappel and Klastersky 1972, Craig and Nahmias 1973). This suggests that type 2 HVH is the predominant cause of herpetic meningitis. Even before direct evidence of the etiologic relation between type 2 HVH and herpetic meningitis was obtained, there were several observations that clearly, in retrospect, hinted that this must be the case. In 1955, Hunt and Comer isolated a strain of herpesvirus from both cerebrospinal fluid and genital tract of patients with meningitis. It is quite conceivable that the virus they isolated was identical with type 2 HVH. The recovery of type 2 HVH from the cerebrospinal fluid (Skoldenberg 1972; Stadler et al. 1973) strongly supports the hypothesis that this agent is a cause of aseptic meningitis. However, there have been several cases of meningitis described in association with gingivostomatitis. This suggests that type 1 HVH may also be capable of producing aseptic meningitis (Brunell and Dodd 1964). In two patients with aseptic meningitis, Sawanobori et al. (1974) succeded in identifying the HVH as type 1 by microneutralization and kinetic-neutralization tests and neutralization tests with type-specific hyperimmune IgM antibodies in the presence of complement.

In general, aseptic meningitis usually develops shortly after the appearance of herpetic lesions, which cannot be demonstrated in about 50 percent of cases. During the acute phase of the illness the cerebrospinal fluid invariably shows pleocytosis, mostly on account of lymphocytes. Protein levels may vary from 50 to 100 mg per 100 ml, whereas sugar levels are within normal ranges.

In contrast to herpetic encephalitis, herpetic meningitis is a rather benign disease characterized by the absence of stupor, convulsions or focal neurologic findings. The patients usually recover completely within a month, but occasionally the disease may assume a recurrent character (Janbon et al. 1942; Duxbury and Lawrence 1959; Terni et al. 1971). Tamalet (1935) has described a case with 17 recurrences of genital herpes associated with meningitis over a period of 14 years.

II. Herpetic encephalitis

In 1933, Dawson reported the finding of intranuclear inclusion bodies within neurons and glial cells of a patient with rapidly progressing and fatal encephalitis. In 1941, Smith *et al.* identified intranuclear inclusion bodies in nerve cells and isolated HVH from the brain of a newborn infant who died of acute encephalitis. Several years later, Coons *et al.* (1950) developed a fluorescent antibody technique for the localization of virus particles in tissue cells. In 1964, MacCallum *et al.* isolated HVH in brain biopsy of two patients with encephalitis.

Herpetic encephalitis seems to be one of the most frequent acute viral infections of the brain in the United States today (Nolan *et al.* 1970; Crausaz 1972; Price *et al.* 1973). It appears to be more frequent than encephalitises resulting from infection with some other viruses including mumps, influenza viruses, Coxackie viruses and ECHO viruses. Gostling (1967) states that HVH accounts for 5—7 percent of viral encephalitises, whereas from the reports of other authors it appears that it may account for 2—20 percent (Lennette *et al.* 1962; Ryden *et al.* 1965; Cappel and Klastersky 1972).

Herpetic encephalitis may develop as a result of either primary or recurrent (or reactivated latent) infection (Good and Campbell 1945; Ginder and Whorten 1951; Leider *et al.* 1965; Gostling 1967; Lizer and Ionnides 1971).

The *pathogenesis* of the disease depends upon the direct cytotoxic (cytopathic) effect of the virus on the one hand, and upon the immune capabilities of the host on the other. Perhaps this might explain the wide variety of clinical features of the disease. It might also be an answer to the question of why herpesvirus sometimes causes only a mild local infection, and sometimes fatal encephalitis (Yamamoto *et al.* 1965). The conditions which may enable the development of herpetic encephalitis in adults have been outlined by Wilt *et al.* (1969).

A. *The virulence of the virus at the time of exposure*

1. The virus is *avirulent* (non-neurotropic). Following a primary exposure, a mild local disease may develop and a subclinical infection of the salivary glands may result (Kaufman *et al.* 1967). During a recurrent attack, the virus may become neurotropic and may ascend via sensory nerves to the central nervous system (Paine 1964; Johnson and Mims 1968).

2. The virus is *virulent* (neurotropic). An initially mild local disease may be followed by the development of chronic subclinical infection that may be activated at a later date and lead to encephalitis. A neurovirulent virus can initially produce a mild upper respiratory infection and ascend the olfactory route (Johnson 1964a, b) to cause encephalitis without inducing an apparent superficial lesion (Rawls 1966; Olson *et al.* 1967).

B. *Immune status of the host*

1. In persons lacking specific antibodies a mild local infection or a severe encephalitis may result depending on the virus's virulence.

2. In persons possessing specific antibodies, antibodies to HVH are not entirely effective in preventing infection. This is evidenced by the common knowledge that individuals who have specific antibodies to HVH suffer from recurrent attacks of herpes labialis. The development of herpetic encephalitis in individuals with labial herpes seems to be best explained by assuming that encephalitis results from the introduction of an exogenous neurotropic strain or alternatively that it results from the reactivation of a virulent endogenous strain during one of the recurrent attacks.

3. In persons with secondary immunodeficiencies associated with leukemia, Hodgkin's disease or multiple myeloma, primary infection may on occasion result in severe secondary infections such as disseminated herpes (Price *et al.* 1973).

Until recently the neural route was considered to be the primary if not the sole pathway by which HVH reached the central nervous system (Goodpasture and Teague 1923; Marinesco and Draganesco 1923; Johnson 1964a, b). However, recent experimental work with polioviruses and arboviruses has indicated that viruses can spread to the brain by olfactory or hematogenous routes as well. Spreading along nerves can be either by way of endoneural and perineural cells or by rapid diffusion without apparent cellular involvement. Spreading across the olfactory mucosa can occur either by way of endoneural and perineural cells or by direct infection of the adjacent arachnoid. Infection via the olfactory route could perhaps offer an explanation of the orbital-frontal and temporal lobe localization of encephalitises.

As regards the hematogenous route to the central nervous system, several mechanisms have been postulated (Johnson and Mims 1968; Colonnello and Signorini 1972). It has been suggested that the virus first multiplies in extraneural cells and, if a viremia of sufficient magnitude and duration is established, spreads from small cerebral vessels into the cerebrospinal fluid or directly into the brain tissue. Some viruses can invade the central nervous system by forcing their way through vascular endothelium whereas others can do so by getting carried across the blood brain barrier.

That viruses can spread to the central nervous system by neural, olfactory or hematogenous routes has been demonstrated by antigen tracing studies (Rawls 1966; Johnson and Mims 1968; Price *et al.* 1973). It is clear, however, that the mode of spreading may vary with different viruses, different hosts and different portals of entry.

Different cells of the central nervous system show selective vulnerability to infection with herpesvirus. Accordingly, the effect of infection varies from cell to cell.

Herpesvirus causes a progressively severe derangement of the neurons. At first it alters membrane function as is manifested by stimulus sensitive myoclonus and seizure activity and finally leads to partial or complete paralysis. The virus commonly affects the cerebral cortex, resulting in disorders of perception and memory (parietal and temporal cortex) and of judgment (frontal cortex). Signs of brain stem involvement are also common (oculomotor signs, palsies of cranial nerves); (Dayan *et al.* 1972). Finally, parenchymal necrosis and edema may lead to signs of herniation mimicking an expanding process. Dystonia, tremor and rigidity are also frequently present (Meyer *et al.* 1970). Whenever focal neurologic disturbances associated with convulsions appear at the beginning of a febrile disease presenting the *clinical picture* of an encephalitis, serious consideration should be given to the possibility that herpesvirus is the causative agent (Adams and Jennett 1967; Hader *et al.* 1967; Wilt *et al.* 1969; Meyer *et al.* 1970).

The onset of herpetic encephalitis is often marked by influenza-like prodromal symptoms of fever, headache and drowsiness. During this period a mucocutaneous eruption may appear. Symptoms reflecting involvement of the central nervous system are prominent: they consist of stiffness in the neck with early deterioration of the sensorium and focal neurologic disorders (cranial nerve palsies, focal seizures and paralysis of upper motor neurons). Specific symptoms (dysphasia, psychomotor disturbances and olfactory hallucinations) that are predominantly unilateral at the beginning of the illness indicate that temporal and orbital regions are heavily affected (Drachman and Adams 1962; Olson *et al.* 1967). These signs are frequently interpreted as indicating an expanding process and surgery is undertaken (Cappel and Klastersky

1972). The increase in intracranial pressure may result in the herniation of cerebellar tonsils. Death usually occurs in the second or third week of the illness. Of patients who survive, the great majority face permanent physical and mental handicap; complete recovery is very rare (Booth *et al.* 1961; Page *et al.* 1967; Hanshaw 1969; Meyer *et al.* 1970; Bligh *et al.* 1972; Crousaz 1972; Haynes 1973).

Thorough examination of patients presenting acute encephalitis is urgent and has a twofold aim; first, exclusion of other causes such as subdural, epidural, or intracerebral abscess, hematoma or tumors (MacCallum *et al.* 1964; Pierce *et al.* 1964; Blackweed *et al.* 1966; Adams and Jennett 1967; Nolan *et al.* 1970; Oxbury and MacCallum 1973); second the definitive diagnosis of herpetic encephalitis.

The *diagnosis* should be based on a fairly typical clinical picture and various laboratory tests; reliable *laboratory evidence* of primary herpesvirus infection is the demonstration of a rising serum antibody titer during the illness. Antibodies formed in response to primary infection appear in the serum by the end of the first week, reach a maximum titer in the third week of illness and then gradually disappear (Thieffry *et al.* 1955). It is therefore recommended that serial serum samples be taken from each patient suspected of encephalitis. Ross and Stevenson (1961) and some other workers in the field have proposed that a fourfold or greater rise in serum antibody titer be taken as indicative of a current herpesvirus infection. Miller and Ross (1968) claim that a single titer should be greater than 1 in 512, whereas Gostling (1967) thinks it justifiable to accept a fourfold rise of a titer of 160 or more as evidence of active herpetic infection.

Examination of cerebrospinal fluid invariably shows moderate pleocytosis, primarily due to lymphocytes. Many authors have pointed out that the finding of red blood cells in spinal fluid is characteristic of herpetic encephalitis (Booth *et al.* 1961; Rawls 1966; Hanshaw 1969; Haynes 1973; Price *et al.* 1973). Protein concentrations may be normal at the beginning, but as the disease progresses the levels increase (Hanshaw 1969; Haynes 1973). Isolation of the virus from cerebrospinal fluid by direct inoculation of the material into cell cultures of fibroblasts, human amnion, rhesus-monkey kidney or chorioallantoic membrane of embryonated egg has also been tried, but with little success.

Abnormal *electroencephalographic patterns* may offer a clue to the diagnosis of herpetic encephalitis. Most workers agree that serial EEG records that show rapid development of periodic complexes superimposed on a diffuse slow-wave background during the early phase of the illness (2—15 days), followed by disappearance of these complexes without parallel clinical improvement, may be considered diagnostic of herpesvirus encephalitis (Meyer *et al.* 1970; Scott and Prior 1970; Upton and Gumpert 1970; Upton *et al.* 1971; Dayan *et al.* 1972; Illis and Taylor 1972).

Isotope encephalography may also be taken as a guide to the extent of CNS involvement. The results of brain scanning in patients with herpetic encephalitis show that the temporal lobes are most commonly affected though discrete areas of isotope uptake in other parts of the brain may also be found (Castleman 1964; Breeden *et al.* 1966; Balfour *et al.* 1967; Page *et al.* 1967; McKee 1968; Bligh *et al.* 1972). Thus, it has been reported that brain scans may reveal multifocal and asymmetric localization of the isotope (Meyer *et al.* 1970), or patchy areas of focal uptake, or resemble the doughnut appearance characteristic of brain abscesses (Haynes 1973). In one of the reported cases of herpes encephalitis, brain scan revealed the lesion adjacent to the cranial vault and resembling a subdural hematoma (Page *et al.* 1967). There is evidence to suggest that the reason for the increased isotope uptake in cases of herpes encephalitis is severe localized destruction of the brain tissue.

In patients with negative brain scans, further neuroradiologic investigations will most probably fail to show evidence of central nervous system involvement in this disease (Amin 1972). Some workers maintain that in about one-half of the patients presenting acute herpesvirus encephalitis (acute necrotizing encephalitis) the diagnosis can be established by angiography on the basis of characteristic unilateral changes in the temporal lobe region (Döpper and Spaar 1971). One of the most frequently described findings is displacement of the middle cerebral artery with elevation of its proximal portion which resembles the course observed in the presence of a space-occupying lesion.

Although neuroradiologic findings are in themselves non specific, they nevertheless may contribute to the diagnosis by indicating the need for *brain biopsy* and thus lead to a firm diagnosis. There can be little doubt that brain biopsy made through a temporal burr hole is most helpful for the rapid confirmation of the diagnosis. The biopsy specimen can be used for direct viral cultures, for the demonstration of intranuclear inclusion bodies and for the immunofluorescent detection of herpesvirus antigens (Hanshaw 1969; Dayan *et al.* 1972; Haynes 1973).

On microscopic examination the biopsy specimen reveals infiltration of lymphocytes, proliferation of astrocytes and focal perivascular hemorrhages (Haymaker *et al.* 1959; Booth *et al.* 1961; Drachman and Adams 1962; Meyer *et al.* 1970; Rappel *et al.* 1971). The arachnoid over the affected area shows fibrinocellular exudate consisting primarily of mononuclear cells. Many ganglion cells, oligodendroglia and astrocytes are found to contain Cowdry type A inclusions consisting of acidophilic, homogeneous intranuclear structures that are frequently separated from the nuclear membrane by a clear halo (Smith *et al.* 1941; Haymaker 1949; Hader *et al.* 1967; Rappel *et al.* 1971; Dubois-Dalcq *et al.* 1972). These findings are characteristic though nonspecific, but in association with necrotic lesions in patients with acute encephalitis they can be considered diagnostic of herpesvirus infection (Booth *et al.* 1961). Attempts to isolate the virus from brain tissue have included direct inoculation of the biopsy material into cell cultures of human amnion, rhesus-monkey kidney, or chorioallantoic membrane of chick embryo, or into newborn mice, in which the virus produces a typical cytopathic effect (Fingerland and Toušek 1950; Kerenyi *et al.* 1959; Wilt *et al.* 1969; Rappel *et al.* 1971). In positive cultures strain identification is proved by neutralization tests with specific herpesvirus antisera (Dayan *et al.* 1972). Attempts to grow the virus may be variably successful depending on its distribution in the brain tissue.

From the pathologic point of view, herpesvirus affects both gray and white matter and procudes an encephalitis with necrosis, edema and softening (Fig. 15). Although the temporal and insular regions are most consistently involved, the hippocampus cingulate gyrus, orgital surface of the frontal lobe, parietal and occipital cortex, basal ganglia and hypothalamus may also be affected (Haymaker *et al.* 1958; Booth *et al.* 1961; Bellanti *et al.* 1968; Johnson and Olson 1969; Hughes 1969; Radcliffe *et al.* 1971; Crausaz 1972; Illis and Taylor 1972).

Nolan *et al.* (1970) have proposed the following criteria for diagnosis:

(1) a clinical picture of encephalitis with abnormal electroencephalogram.

(2) cerebrospinal fluid sterile for bacteria (including Mycobacterium tuberculosis), and viruses other than HVH.

(3) exclusion of a diagnosis of subdural, epidural or intracerebral abscess, hematoma or tumor by craniotomy.

(4) fourfold rise in serum antibody titer to HVH.

(5) isolation of HVH from brain biopsy or at autopsy.

However, histologic examination of brain tissue can never be more than suggestive, and may show only nonspecific features. Electron microscope demonstration of the virus in tissue seems difficult for routine purposes (Harland *et al.* 1967). Isolation of the virus in culture should be more satisfactory, but it involves a delay of at least 36—48 hours. Antibody changes in the serum or cerebrospinal fluid are necessarily late and in any case the results are variable (Johnson *et al.* 1968; Gilbert *et al.* 1972). For speed the method of choice may well become immunofluorescent demonstration of viral antigen, either in brain-biopsy specimens or perhaps in cells from cerebrospinal fluid (Dayan and Stokes 1973; Nahmias *et al.* 1974) but only when the technique has become reliable.

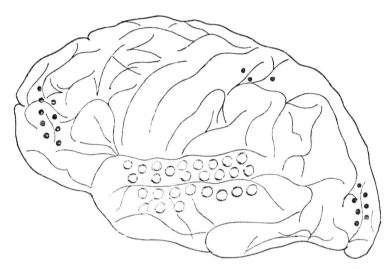

Fig. 15. Sites of major pathology in herpes simplex encephalitis (Illi*s* and Taylor 1972).

III. Prognosis and therapy

The ultimate prognosis of herpes virus encephalitis in terms of mortality and incidence of sequelae is bad even though these have varied in different series. Thus, Leider *et al.* (1965) describe a series of 15 patients of whom 4 died, 3 required permanent institutional care, 2 had memory losses, 1 had hemiparesis with severe behavioral problems and 5 survived without apparent sequelae. Olson *et al.* (1967) report a series of 36 patients of whom 25 died and 3 survived without sequelae. In the series presented by Miller *et al.* (1966) the mortality rate was 50 percent (10 of 20 patients), but only 3 of the 13 who experienced coma and convulsions survived. McKee (1968) states that the mortality rate is about 80 percent in untreated patients. Nolan *et al.* (1970) conclude that patients who are in coma or suffer from convulsions have a poor prognosis. According to their experience, the mortality rate is about 60 percent among untreated patients.

Most workers have emphasized that treatment of patients with herpetic encephalitis should be initiated as early as possible, preferably within the first 48 hours if therapy is to be successful. Implementation is difficult because, in the early phase, the majority of patients do not show symptoms that would justify brain biopsy (Haymaker *et al.* 1959; Marshall 1967; Nolan *et al.* 1970; Silk and Roome 1970; Jelić *et al.* 1973).

Several authors have suggested that many of the severe neurologic sequelae or the death of patients with herpetic encephalitis are more the result of cerebral edema, intracranial pressure and tentorial herniation than of irreversible neuronal damage (Grant and McMenemey 1959; Woolfe and Hoult 1961; Marshall 1967; Page *et al.* 1967). Accordingly, many workers believe that *early and extensive frontotemporo-parietal decompressive craniotomy* may increase the chance of survival (Marshall 1967; Rappel *et al.* 1971). If increased intracranial pressure or clinical deterioration persists it is advisable to perform decompression of the opposite cerebral hemisphere and to apply other supportive measures such as "*medical decompression*" with mannitol, glycerol or hypertonic urea. In such situations, administration of steroids seems to be contraindicated (Page *et al.* 1967; Upton *et al.* 1971). Although the use of ACTH and corticosteroids remains to some extent controversial (Longson and Beswick 1971; Cappel and Klastersky 1972), "medical decompression" may well be as good as surgical decompression (Page *et al.* 1967; Upton *et al.* 1971; Illis and Taylor 1972). Tokumaru (1963, 1968), studying experimentally induced herpes encephalitis in guinea pigs, demonstrated that cortisone did not significantly change the survival time of his animals. This is in agreement with the clinical results reported by Evans *et al.* (1967), Silk and Roome (1970), Upton and Gumpert (1970), and Illis and Taylor (1972).

Within the past few years, favorable therapeutic results have, been reported with *5-iodo-2-deoxyuridine* -IDU (Nolan *et al.* 1973), a drug that is widely used in the treatment of herpetic keratitis (Kaufman 1963; Maxwell 1963). The mechanism by which IDU affects some viruses is based on the inhibition of incorporation of thymide into DNA (Calabresi 1963). Buckley and MacCallum (1967) administered IDU by intracarotid perfusion but without apparent therapeutic effect. At present, most authors recommend intravenous application of IDU at a total dosage of 400—600 mg per kilogram of body weight over a period of 5 to 7 days. During and after IDU therapy it is important to observe the side effects of the drug by regular monitoring of white-blood-cell and platelet counts. Early symptoms of drug toxicity include nausea, vomiting and diarrhea (Meyer *et al.* 1970). Complications of IDU administration include stomatitis, bone marrow depression (leukopenia and thrombocytopenia) and alopecia. However, all these side effects seem to be transient (Meyer et al. 1970; Silk and Roome 1970; Illis and Taylor 1972; Rappel et al. 1971; Longson and Beswick 1971) and thrombocytopenia can be managed by platelet infusion. There have been some reports of a hepatotoxic effect of IDU (Dayan and Lewis 1969; Rappel et al. 1971; Silk and Roome 1970; Rappel 1971).

More recently, therapeutic trials have been made with *cytosine arabinoside (ara-C)* a potent inhibitor of DNA viruses (McKelvey and Kwaan 1969; Juel-Jensen 1970; Price et al. 1973). It has been recommended that the drug be administered intrathecally in a daily dose of 2—3 mg per kilogram of body weight over a period of 4 to 5 days. In contrast to IDU, cytosine arabinoside (ara-C) seems to be less effective across the blood-brain barrier. Women in child bearing age should be given this drug with caution because it may induce trisomy at group C. Symptoms of drug toxicity include nausea, vomiting, leukopenia and thrombocytopenia. There have been some reports that interferon-inducers might also be of therapeutic help (Bellanti et al. 1971). Sidwell et al. (1968) report on a very interesting new antiviral compound called *adenine arabinoside or vidarabine (ara-A)*, a purine nucleoside active against DNA-viruses, which looks like one of the most promising substances for the treatment of neonatal HVH infections, with no apparent toxicity to the bone marrow, liver, or kidney (see also Chapter 16).

There can be no question, however, that none of the drugs thus far tried has proved to be unequivocally efficient in combating herpesvirus infections. Nevertheless, as Hanshaw (1969) said: "We are rapidly approaching a period in which several antiviral substances are reaching a stage in development where trials in human beings with certain life-threatening viral diseases may be justified. The rapid expansion of knowledge of the phases in the viral replicative sequence, the recognition of the important differences between the metabolic requirements of the virus and host cells and the encouraging results in animal systems should give the clinician hope that therapy with antiviral, as well as antibacterial drugs may at least be pharmacologically feasible. Although there are major obstacles ahead such as serious drug toxicity, possible development of viral resistance and the teratogenic effects of powerful DNA inhibitors, the prospects for future successful systemic therapy seem a step closer to realization."

Chapter 10

HERPESVIRUS AND SOME NEUROPSYCHIATRIC DISORDERS

Herpesvirus is presently recognized as an etiologic agent in acute diseases of the central nervous system, causing encephalitis and aseptic meningitis in all age groups. The type 1 HVH strain is usually responsible for encephalitis.

Several authors have suggested that HVH may play a role in subacute and chronic diseases of the central nervous system in man. In 1964 Gudnadottir et al. reported the isolation of HVH from the brain of a patient with *multiple sclerosis*. The virus was subsequently shown to be a type 2 strain (Nahmias and Dowdle 1968). Neutralization studies of serum from 53 Icelandic multiple-sclerosis patients revealed that 96 percent had antibodies to this virus whereas fewer than 70 percent of control sera neutralized the virus. A somewhat poorer correlation between two groups had been found in Great Britain and Belgium (Gudnadottir et al. 1964). Some other studies have confirmed these findings, showing higher levels of herpetic antibodies in the serum of patients with multiple sclerosis than in the control sera (Plummer and Hackett 1966, Ortona et al. 1972). Catalano (1972) reports that his patients with multiple sclerosis appeared to have moderate elevations of antibody levels to type 2 HVH, whereas no increased antibody levels to type 1 were detected.

Other surveys of serum and cerebrospinal fluid for elevated complement fixing antibody titers to herpesvirus revealed no differences between multiple sclerosis patients and controls (Reed et al. 1964; Ross et al. 1965, 1969; Terni and Luzzatto 1969). The results of these investigations are completely negative with respect to isolation and serology of both types of herpesvirus.

In a recent study by Brody et al. (1971), virus antibody titers of multiple sclerosis patients were found higher than titers of carefully matched controls for measles, type C influenza, herpesvirus, parainfluenza 3, mumps and varicella-zoster, and not consistently higher than titers of controls for adenovirus, parainfluenza 1 and types A and B influenza. Virus antibody titers to any of these agents were not higher among multiple sclerosis patients than were titers of their siblings. This finding suggested a familial factor in these responses (Brody *et al.* 1971).

Plummer *et al.* (1968) examined 9 sera from patients with *amyotrophic lateral sclerosis* and found neutralizing antibody levels to HVH that were fourfold to eightfold the levels found in any of the 50 control sera from a similar age group. These elevated antibody levels were against the type 1 strain. No significant elevations of type specific HVH antibodies to either strain of the virus were detected in the serum of patients with amyotrophic lateral sclerosis in the study by Catalano (1971).

Involvement of the CNS with the clinical picture of *cerebellar ataxia* is reported by Dano (1968). It is described in an 8-year old boy who had simultaneous herpetic gingivitis. Primary herpetic infection was confirmed by serologic tests.

The first case of *myelitis ascendens* etiologically associated with herpes was reported by Craig and Nahmias (1971). They isolated HVH type 2 from a genital lesion; culture of the cerebrospinal fluid for the virus was negative. The same disease with a fulminant clinical course was published by Klastersky *et al.* (1972). They isolated HVH type 1 from the cerebrospinal fluid.

A preliminary report by Nishimura (1973) suggests that the virus associated with subacute *myelopticoneuropathy* is possibly a new member of the herpes virus group, although its type-specific neutralizing antigen is quite different from that of types 1 and 2.

Further investigation is needed to establish the possible etiologic role of herpesviruses in all these neurologic disorders.

Although the clinical differences between zoster and herpes simplex are often unmistakable, they are not always so. Several cases of *zoster-like disease* have been caused by the virus of herpes simplex.

In his original studies of herpes zoster Lipschütz (1921) described two cases from which he succesfully transferred the infectious agent to the cornea of rabbits (cit. by Slavin and Ferguson 1950). The first instances of the isolation of herpesvirus from zoster-like eruption of the face were reported by Teague and Goodpasture (1923) and Freund (1928).

Slavin and Ferguson (1950) collected from the literature 16 cases of zoster-like eruption in man, from which herpesvirus was isolated by transfer to the cornea of rabbits. They also added 5

cases of their own with zoster-like eruptions where similar transfer of the infectious agent to animals was successful. In addition,
specific HVH antibodies were found in the serum. The fifth of these
cases, in a 6-year-old boy, was probably not zoster. Four days
after admission he developed aphthous stomatitis, perioral herpes
and painful swelling of the right middle finger. This was a typical
example of autoinoculation.

Ragazzini (1962) describes a very instructive case in a 4-year-old
girl, who developed some recurrences of zosterlike eruptions on
the right side of the face, neck, and the right arm during the course
of tuberculous meningitis. The girl had a history of probable primary
herpetic infection in the mouth when 18 months old. HVH was
isolated from the vesicles.

In the report by Slavin and Ferguson (1950) the trigeminal
area was involved in 4 of the 21 patients. In one patient the dermal
manifestations were preceded or accompanied by neuralgic pain.
Three additional cases of recurrent herpes simplex of the face associated with neuralgia were reported by Behrman and Knight
(1954). Stroud (1961) has published a case of a patient with primary
amyloidosis who had a recurrent zoster-like herpes simplex infection
of the sacral region. Tanaka and Southam (1965) found that the
injection of HVH into newborn mice resulted in a segmental infection
of the animals quite similar to the segmental lesions of herpes zoster
in man.

A similar case with burning pain followed by a herpetic rash
along the sciatic nerve — *herpetic sciatica* — was described by
Siegel (1969), but unfortunately no biologic or serologic confirmation
was obtained.

A very interesting report by Music et al. (1971) describes a rare
zosteriform eruption in a newborn from whom HVH was isolated.

Cushing (1905, cited by Constantine et al. 1968) was the first
to describe *herpetiform lesions following section of the trigeminal nerve
for neuralgia*. This correlation was subsequently confirmed (Carton
and Kilbourne 1952). Constantine et al. (1968) reported a 46-year-old
man, who had recurrent herpes simplex on the forehead associated
with neuralgia and regional adenopathy. The pain preceded the skin
lesions by about 24 hours. Herpesvirus was isolated from the lesions
and identified.

Recently experimental zosteriform herpes simplex infection
was produced in mouse skin (Robinson and Dover 1972). HVH has
been isolated from the trigeminal ganglia in rabbits (Nesburn et
al. 1972) and in man (Baringer and Swoveland 1973).

It is not known what strain of HVH is mainly responsible for
zoster-like eruptions or by what mechanism peripheral-nerve lesions
activate latent herpes simplex skin infections.

Final confirmation of the hypothesis that *Bell's palsy* may be caused by HVH infection must await a careful prospective attempt to isolate HVH from the affected nerve (McCormick 1972). The finding of complement-fixing antibodies to HVH in 100 percent of adult patients with idiopathic facial paralysis in the series of Adour *et al.* (1975) does not confirm etiologic association because of the high prevalence of antibodies in the normal adult population. A rise in antibody titer indicating primary herpetic infection was not found in these patients.

Several papers have suggested that herpesvirus infection may be associated *with psychiatric disorders*. For example, Rimon and Halonen (1969) reported that 28 psychotic depressives showed higher complement fixation titers against HVH than did other psychiatric patients and non-psychiatric persons. In the study by Cleobury and Skinner (1971) serum samples from a small series of patients were examined for HVH antibody and an unusually high average kinetic neutralization constant against type 1 herpesvirus was found in the group of aggressive psychopaths, whereas a fivefold lower level of antibodies was found in other general hospital patients. A leading article in the *British Medical Journal* (1971) also supports the working hypothesis of a virus infection during childhood (either inapparent or at least unrecognized) that damages frontotemporal areas of the brain related to personality.

The association of HVH and psychiatric disorders still requires further investigations using more rigorously defined control groups and other virus antigens.

Chapter 11

HERPETIC DISEASE OF THE EYE

V. RIBARIĆ

Herpetic keratitis presents a special problem among clinical eye diseases both as regards the course of the disease and treatment. It is a frequent and widespread disease representing, according to some authors, the commonest virus infection of the human eye and, according to Nataf *et al.* (1960), contributing 20 percent of all eye pathology.

It is caused by herpesvirus hominis (HVH), a ubiquitous virus that latently lives its saprophytic life on visible human mucous membranes or in other foci of the organism (Frezzotti and Guerra 1971).

Herpetic disease of the cornea was first reported by Horner (in 1870, cit. by Frezzotti and Guerra, 1971). Grüter (1920) first succeeded in infecting the cornea of a rabbit by HVH causing the same symptoms as those in man. He was convinced that it was an infectious disease produced by HVH. Then he transferred the infection from the eye to the cornea of a blind man; a typical form of the disease developed. The virus shows special tropism for mucocutaneous localizations (dermatotropism) and nerve tissue (neurotropism). The high frequency of herpetic eye disease caused by HVH today can be explained by the reduction in microbic disease as a result of antibiotic therapy, greater numbers of people, improved means of transportation, great contagiousness of the virus, a lack of specific drugs and various other factors. The disease is the more dangerous because it attacks all ages and both sexes. The consequences can be very different ranging from complete recovery to loss of eyesight. Inflammation of the iris of the involved eye, very often pussy and hemorrhagic, of the ciliary body and both complications together are observed in severe cases (Cavara and Bietti 1952; Witmer and Inomato 1968; Thygeson and Kimura 1957; Kaufman *et al.* 1971). Some rare cases of herpetic chorioretinitis have also been reported (Battignani 1934; Bobo 1970;

Laibson 1970). At present, some 70-90 percent of the whole population is considered to be infected by HVH. Nevertheless, many who are infected never suffer from herpetic keratitis, so that infection does not necessarily lead to an eye infection.

One can come into contact with HVH even during one's first appearance in the world, that is, at the time of delivery, if the mother suffers from genital herpes. The genital source can, rather exceptionally, lead to a primary eye infection, herpetic keratitis, with serious consequences (Bobo *et al.* 1970).

Primary infection very often occurs during infancy and early childhood, but is usually abortive. Herpetic keratitis is more frequent in adults than in children, and in men than in women. Herpetic eye disease, of the cornea especially, mostly involves only one eye, during the period of onset, only very rarely both of them at the same time. Gundersen (1936) found only one bilateral herpetic keratitis in a series of 221 clinical cases. Thygeson and Kimura (1957) had 19 cases of bilateral herpetic keratitis among 200 patients. Stanković and Dučić-Petrović (1964) report 5 out of 76 cases. Ribarić (1968) found none in 185 cases. Klinger (1969) reports none in a series of 61 children. Generally speaking, herpetic keratitis has a dominant place among corneal diseases, especially in its relapsing form.

I Epidemiology

Man is a natural host of herpesvirus being a source of his own infection. Herpetic keratitis is etiologically associated with HVH type 1 infection as it relates to adults, that is, recurrent herpetic keratitis in adults and older children. Type 2 HVH is etiologically associated primarily with human genital herpes, and is considered to be an important cause of primary herpetic keratitis of the newborn (Nahmias and Dowdle 1968; Bobo *et al.* 1970; Proto and Tedesco 1966; Frezzotti and Guerra 1971). According to Nahmias's study of epidemiologic data, herpetic eye disease occurs in 1 out of 3 500 to 30 000 newborns. Social and economic factors are of great importance in the spread of infection. We were not able to find any epidemiologic data in the available literature on the relation between primary and recurrent herpetic infection of the eye. Therefore we shall try to find these data among clinical cases of herpetic keratitis during the follow up period.

It may be generally considered that primary herpetic infection of the eye occurs mainly in children up to the age of 10 and cases of primary herpetic infection in older children and adults are very rare. The incidence of primary herpetic infection can be estimated indirectly, from the number of children up to the age of 10 with herpetic infection in relation to the total number of persons suffering from herpetic keratitis attending clinic during a definite interval of time. Different authors give the percentages of manifest primary herpetic infection in children up to 10 years as listed in Table 1.

Table 1. *Rate of herpetic disease among children hospitalized on eye wards*

Author	Period of observation (years)	Percentage with herpetic eye disease
Blagojević and Ilić (1964)	14	6
Stanković and Dučić-Petrović (1964)	9	13
Klinger (1969)	10	18
Talanyi-Pfeifer (1972)	5	6

According to these findings *manifest primary eye infection occurs in between 6 and 18*, in an average of 11 percent of children up to age 10.

The incidence of recurrent disease has been estimated from the number of cases of herpetic keratitis with one or more relapses within 2 years occurring in patients of 10 years old or older, as follows: Carroll *et al.* (1967) 43 percent; Jawetz *et al.* (1970) 40 percent; and Frezzotti and Guerra (1971) 40 percent. This gives an average incidence of 42 percent among adults. The ratio of recurrent to primary infection from the above figures is 42:12 or approximately 4:1.

According to many authors herpetic keratitis very often appears in dendritic form during clinical study within a definite period of time (Table 2).

The sequelae rate of all forms of herpetic keratitis, especially of the two most frequent, is about 22 percent. This refers to type 1 HVH. The recurrence of type 2 HVH cannot be ascertained exactly, but is probably less than 1:4 (the ratio of primary to recurrent disease) since type 2 HVH occurs as a primary infection from mothers genitally infected with type 2 HVH only in a small number of newborns.

Table 2. *The occurrence of different forms of herpetic keratitis*

Keratitis dendritica	Percent	Keratitis disciformis	Percent
Author Blagojević and Ilić (1964)	76	Author Blagojević and Ilić (1964)	25
Stanković and Dučić-Petrović (1964)	84	Stanković and Dučić-Petrović (1964)	10
Ribarić (1968)	84	Ribarić (1968)	22
Klinger (1969)	70	Thygeson (1967)	10
Talanyi-Pfeifer (1972)	79		

It seems probable that the incidence of herpetic keratitis differs among different population groups, in different countries and on different continents (Coetze 1955) but we have no data on this.

II Clinical picture

Primary herpetic eye infection of the newborn can occur during delivery by a mother suffering from manifest herpetic vulvovaginitis, but it is very rare (Zuelzer and Stulberg 1952; Battignani 1934; Bobo *et al.* 1970; Frezzotti and Guerra 1971; Cibis and Burde 1971). The disease is most frequent during early infancy after the sixth month because the baby is transplacentally protected by the mother's specific herpetic antibodies up to this time. It may also occur in later childhood (at school or boarding school) because of the crowding of contacts (Nahmias *et al.* 1968; Hagler *et al.* 1969; Juretić and Petković 1960; Klinger 1969; Proto and Tedesco 1966; Stanković and Dučić-Petrović 1964). Primary herpetic infection attacks both sexes, and can involve almost all eye structures and tanexa: the skin and border of the eyelids (blepharitis herpetica vesiculosa) — a disease of benign course, without consequences on eye function; — the *conjunctiva* (conjunctivitis herpetica follicularis) predominantly involving conjunctiva of the fornix with preauricalular adenopathy; — the *cornea* (keratitis herpetica punctata superficialis), without involving a corneal stroma, in principle, without corneal scars; — the *cornea and conjunctiva* (keratoconjunctivitis herpetica), the most frequent form of herpetic primary infection of the human eye, which can exist by itself or in association with herpetic infection of the skin or mucosa or with visceral herpetic lesions; — the *choroidea* and *retina* (chorioretinitis herpetica), a form of the disease that is seldom met (Frezzotti and Guerra 1971; Howard 1966; Kimura 1963; White *et al.* 1968), — encephalitis, a rare but often lethal disease (Ribarić and Batistić 1973).

Relapsing or *recurrent herpetic eye disease* — is any such disease that recurs at the place of primary infection. Recurrence is demonstrated by finding specific herpetic antibodies in the blood of the patient on the first day of onset (Frezzotti and Guerra 1971; Blank and Rake 1955; Carrol *et al.* 1967; Kaufman *et al.* 1967). A relapse means not reinfection but reactivation of a latent virus in the organism after primary herpetic infection (Scott and Tokumaru 1964). Reactivation follows various provocative factors such as trauma, fever, menses, emotional stress, anaphylaxis, local administration of corticosteroids (Kaufman 1963), weakening of local immunity (Scalise *et al.* 1970), and others. Fever, trauma and emotional stress are most common in clinical practice. A latent virus may be present in the form of a non infectious "provirus" subdued, to provocative factors, or it may be in an infectious form remaining latent in a labile balance with specific antibodies in the organism, also subdued: to provocative factors from within or without (Hanna *et al.* 1957; Thygeson and Kimura 1957; Kaufman *et al.* 1968). Because of the presence of antibodies the avascular cornea is considered to be more frequently involved by relapsing herpetic keratitis than the vascular conjunctiva (Thygeson and Kimura 1957).

Recurrent herpetic disease is usually characterized by different types of corneal involvement (Frezzotti and Guerra 1971) although the iris and ciliary body may be involved (Kimura 1963; Kaufman *et al.* 1971; Saraux 1966; Witmer and Inomato 1968), and disease of the optic nerve has been observed (Cavara and Bietti 1952).

The course of recurrent herpetic keratitis depends on such factors as virulence of the virus, type of lesion, environment, therapy applied and duration of the disease before treatment. In principle, the disease is curable. Recurrent herpetic keratitis may have:

(1) early recurrence, within a few weeks of the previous herpetic illness (Klinger 1969). The reason for the early relapse has to be investigated; one must look into such things as inadequate therapy, the immunologic condition of the organism and provocative factors from without and within.

(2) late recurrences, from a few months several years after a previous herpetic infection (Sexton 1970; Nataf *et al.* 1960; Hughes W. F., 1969).

II Classification of disease and clinical forms

There are different forms of herpetic keratitis in the group of primary infection and early and late recurrences of the disease, differing morphologically from one another, and several attempts have been made to classify them:

(1) Thygeson and Kimura (1957)
  (a) surface keratitis
  (b) deep keratitis

(2) Velhagen and Sorby, 1964 (cit. by Frezzotti and Guerra, 1971)
  (a) epithelial keratitis
  (b) parenchymatous keratitis
  (c) endothelial keratitis

(3) Frezzotti and Guerra (1971)
  (a) surface initial keratitis
  (b) surface progressive keratitis
  (c) deep keratitis (disciform)
  (d) deep keratitis involving the epithelium
  (e) deep keratitis involving the anterior eye segment
     (Laibson 1970).

In spite of their practical value, these classifications are not completely satisfactory because of some general principles of classification. Classification should be based on such factors as the clinical form of the disease, the layer of the cornea involved and the progression of the infection. For instance, there are epithelial forms of the disease that remain epithelial throughout. There are mixed forms involving the layer of the cornea adjacent to the epithelial layer and combined with it which give the disease certain characteristics. There are also deep forms that can occur close to or along with the superficial forms. The following classification is based on the above principles.

(4) Ribarić (1976):
  (a) epithelial keratitis (keratitis punctata superficialis)
  (b) epithelial-stromal (ulcera herpetica corneae)
  (c) stromal (keratitis herpetica disciformis)
  (d) stromal-endothelial (progressive keratitis herpetica posterior)
  (e) endothelial (keratitis herpetica posterior)
  (f) stromal, involving deeper eye structures (iritis, iridocyclitis, chorioretinitis herpetica)

The following clinical types of disease can be seen either alone or in combination:

(1) keratoconjunctivitis herpetica
(2) keratitis punctata superficialis
(3) keratitis vesiculosa (Horner 1871, cit. by Frezzotti and Guerra, 1971)
(4) keratitis dendritica (Emmert 1885, cit. by Frezzotti and Guerra, 1971)
(5) keratitis girlandiforme (Ribarić 1973)
(6) keratitis geographica
(7) keratitis stellata
(8) keratitis disciformis (Fuchs 1901, cit. by Frezzotti and Guerra, 1971)
(9) ulcus herpeticum corneae (Grut 1884, cit. by Frezzotti and Guerra, 1971)
(10) keratitis posterior
(11) keratitis herpetica bullosa
(12) keratitis metaherpetica (Gundersen and Bietti 1936)
(13) keratitis et Iridocyclitis herpetica (Cavara and Bietti 1952)
(14) chorioretinitis herpetica (Laibson 1970)

Keratitis herpetica dendritica is the commonest and most typical form of the disease, especially in relapse. It can appear alone or with any other form of the disease and accounts for 75 percent of all clinical types of herpetic keratitis (Pavan-Langston and Mc-Culley 1973; Laibson 1970; Kimura 1963; Klinger 1969; Cavara and Bietti 1952; Doden et al. 1970; Baron et al. 1959).

Keratitis herpetica disciformis is a typical deep form of the disease. It is now considered to be an expression of immunoallergic reaction of the cornea to HVH. It accounts for 10—25 percent of all cases of herpetic keratitis in man. (Blagojević and Ilić 1964; Stanković and Dučić-Petrović 1964; Ribarić 1968; Saraux 1966; Thygeson and Kimura 1957; Offre et al. 1966; Bonamour 1969).

Keratitis metaherpetica is a chronic and serious form of the disease distinguished by some specific characteristics from other forms of herpetic keratitis. Because HVH cannot be isolated from the cornea, and because the disease is therefore considered to be trophic in nature some authors call it keratitis trofica (Gundersen 1936; Bonamour 1969; Nataf et al. 1960; Kimura 1963).

Clinical diagnosis of herpetic keratitis is not difficult if it is manifested by typical herpetic efflorescence of the cornea as is most frequently the case. Sometimes, however, it is not easy to make the diagnosis, in an atypical manifestation of the disease when the differential diagnosis suggests some other disease of the cornea.

Accurate diagnosis of herpetic keratitis can be made by virus isolation (inoculation of an animal cornea or tissue culture) (Grüter 1920; Coleman and Thygeson 1969; Hana 1957), serologic testing (direct and indirect immunofluorescence) proving herpetic antibodies (Kaufman *et al.* 1969; Campinchi *et al.* 1967; Gardner *et al.* 1968; Liotet and Bonnin 1965; Richardson *et al.* 1969; Scalise *et al.* 1970) and, most recently, by microscopy (pathohistologic study of infected cells) demonstrating the typical cytopathogenic effect (Naib *et al.* 1966; Witmer and Inomato 1968).

Each of these methods, with the exception of inoculation of an animal cornea, requires highly technical equipment and professional skill for carrying out a diagnostic test.

IV Therapy

The therapy of herpetic eye disease remains one of the unsolved problems in herpetic disease in general. No therapy for herpetic eye disease, especially herpetic keratitis, is universally successful despite the newer types of treatment that are being reported.

The biologic qualities and the evolutionary cycle of the virus that causes the disease, HVH have to be taken into consideration in our attitude toward this important and responsible task (Scott and Tokumaru 1970).

Present therapy in herpetic keratitis is exclusively local, with the exception of peroral use of broad spectrum antibiotics (Blagojević and Ilić 1964; Stanković and Dučić-Petrović 1964; Kaufman 1963, 1969; Jawetz *et al.* 1970; Abadzhyan *et al.* 1971; Guerra *et al.* 1970; Pavan-Langston and Dohlman 1972; Jawetz 1973).

A recent approach to therapy is directed towards complete inactivation of the latent virus, thus preventing relapses. The technique involves continuous fever therapy for 36-48 hours to produce thermoinactivation of the virus which is known to show thermal sensitivity. Such general fever therapy, without specific local treatment, has given therapeutic results in the treatment of experimental herpetic keratitis in rhesus monkeys (Ribarić 1973).

It has been shown that after an attack of herpetic keratitis, HVH remains latent in the cornea, conjunctiva, adnexa, tear gland and neighboring tissues (Horsfall and Tamm 1970; Kaufman 1970; Sexton 1970; Frezzotti and Guerra 1971). Since the cornea reacts to general fever therapy, thermoinactivation of the latent virus in the eye might be expected to give good therapeutic results (Ribarić 1973).

Therapeutic methods in herpetic keratitis can be divided into several groups:

(1) Various local mechanical, physical and chemical methods used to destroy the infected cell and the virus in it (including operative methods, mechanical and chemical abrasion, X-rays, ultraviolet rays, cold and all kinds of local heat application) (Amman 1946; Cavara and Bietti 1952; Corwin and Tanne 1970; Gomperts 1968; Hughes 1969; Krwawicz 1965, 1968; Offret et al. 1966; Ribarić and Gligo 1972, Ribarić et al. 1971; Segal et al. 1967).

(2) Enzymatic methods, immunization (with vaccine) and other methods to reinforce the immunobiological potential of the organism (Frezzotti and Guerra 1971; Little et al. 1969; Wassermanova and Kubelka 1959; Pouliquen et al. 1966; Scalise et al. 1970; Stock and Aronson 1970).

(3) Chemotherapeutics and antibiotics in local and general administration (Frezzotti and Guerra 1971; Bonamour 1969; Blagojević and Ilić 1964).

(4) Antimetabolites to block the development of the DNA of HVH thus preventing its multiplication (Kaufman et al. 1963, 1969; Carroll et al. 1967; Coleman and Thygeson 1969; Davidson and Evans 1964; Gundersen 1936; Graupner and Muller 1968; Jawetz et al. 1970; Kuchle and Kunze 1964; Park and Baron 1968; Pollikoff et al. 1970.

(5) Interferon and its inducers (poly 1 C) (Abodzyhan et al. 1971, 1968; Cantell and Tommila 1960; Doden 1970; Field et al. 1967; Guerra et al. 1970; Park et al. 1969; Tommila 1963).

(6) Corticosteroids (for deep forms of keratitis) combined with antimetabolites because of their complementary effects (Baron et al. 1959; Kaufman 1963; Saraux 1966).

(7) General continuous pyretic therapy (Ribarić 1973).

(8) Sympathycomimetics (amphetamine) (suggested by Ribarić 1973)

(9) All other therapies (mydriatic, symptomatic, etc.).

The various methods are directed to four different sites:

(1) the cell membrane: bimolin, used locally (Ribarić, 1970)

(2) the cell nucleus: antimetabolites (Kaufman 1963)

(3) the cell metabolism: cold (Krwawicz 1965)

(4) the virus itself, active or latent: general pyretic therapy (Ribarić 1973).

Methods of therapy. In clinical practice therapeutic methods are rarely used singly; they are generally combined. The success of treatment depends on the clinical form of the disease, how far it has progressed before therapy is started and the appropriate combination of therapeutic modalities. The earlier in the disease the therapy is begun the more successful it is likely to be.

Unfortunately, sometimes there are no satisfactory results. Offret *et al.* 1966 (quoted by Frezzotti and Guerra, 1971), rightly say: "With no regard to the therapy applied in herpetic keratitis, there are always individual incurable cases."

V Prognosis

The prognosis in herpetic keratitis varies greatly. There is a significant difference in prognosis between primary infection and the relapsing disease. Generally speaking, the prognosis of primary herpetic eye infection is relatively good, with the exception of some rare forms of herpetic chorioretinitis and cases in which the disease is a manifestation of a generalizing systemic herpetic infection (Battignani 1934; Proto and Tedesco 1966). Prognosis in relapsing herpetic eye disease is relatively unfavorable, because of the serious consequences for eye function from the predominantly involved cornea after every relapse (Saraux 1966; Segal *et al.* 1967; Carol *et al.* 1967; Hana *et al.* 1957; Hughes 1969).

Frequent relapsing herpetic keratitis leads to metaherpetic keratitis (Gundersen 1936). This is the most difficult type of uncomplicated relapsing herpetic keratitis to treat.

Chapter 12

TRAUMATIC HERPES

I Primary traumatic herpes in children

Herpesvirus has a special predilection for mucous membranes and mucocutaneous tissues. There have been many reports of herpetic infection in children occurring in association with constitutional eczema and skin burns. It appears, however, that any lesion on the surface of the skin may become the portal of entry for herpes. Thus Moncrieff observed disseminated herpes on the gluteal skin of an infant with diaper rash (Brain 1956).

Sheward (1961) described primary *perianal herpes* in identical twins with mild diaper rash. The mode of transmission of the virus to the twins is interesting to note. Their father had "cold sores" to which he applied zinc-and-castor-oil ointment. The ointment was also used for treating diaper rashes on the twins. A few days later, typical erythema, vesicles and ulcers developed on the infected areas of both children. Virologic and serologic examinations revealed herpesvirus as the etiologic agent.

It is surprising that perianal and perigenital herpes has not been recognized and described more frequently. Recently, we observed the case of a small child with herpetic eruptions involving a large part of the diaper rash. The infection was most probably transmitted from the child's mother, who had labial herpes at that time. In this case, primary infection was serologically proved (Juretić and Rajh 1976).

Findlay and MacCallum (1940) have described recurrent traumatic herpes in a 2-year-old child with a grazed palm. After the injury, herpetic efflorescences recurred for years on the same area. In their report, Findlay and MacCallum reviewed several cases of recurrent traumatic herpes reported in the literature.

Scott *et al.* (1952) describe recurrent herpes on a burn scar, and Warren and Salvatore (1968) a case of recurrent herpes at the site of smallpox vaccination.

II Herpes gladiatorum

A special form of primary herpes occurring among members of college wrestling teams was first described by Selling and Kibrick in 1964. This form of cutaneous herpes has an epidemic character and occurs as the result of intimate personal contact during wrestling. Herpetic efflorescences consisting of extensive vesicopustular eruptions are usually seen on the right side of the face, and on the scalp, the neck and the flexor surfaces of the arms. These areas of the body are maximally exposed to pressure and abrasion in some wrestling maneuvers ("lock-up" position). In such cases, herpetic lesions usually occur within 7 to 10 days following contact with an infected wrestling mat. Herpes gladiatorum is probably more frequent than is reported. Simple mild forms of the infection are often overlooked.

The diagnosis can be established by virus isolation and serology. In some of the cases reported serologic tests revealed primary infection whereas in others the presence of specific neutralizing antibodies suggested a recurrent herpes resulting most probably from the implantation of the virus through minor lesions or abrasions of the skin. Unfortunately, at the time when such cases were reported, serologic differentiation of the two types of herpesvirus was not performed, and it might be that some of the "recurrent" infections resulted from inoculation with the other type of virus.

Although lesions may often be mistaken for mycotic or bacterial skin infection, it is nevertheless evident that herpes gladiatorum is a not infrequent disease among wrestlers. This is indicated by three independent reports describing similar epidemics of herpesvirus infection among members of different wrestling teams (Wheeler and Cabaniss 1965; Dyke et al. 1965; Porter and Baugham 1965). From the reported observations, it appears that the primary infection is characterized by systemic symptoms, edema of the skin, and regional lymphadenopathy.

The epidemiologic study of Porter and Baugham (1965) indicates that over a 2-year period 84 members of various college wrestling teams in the northeastern United States suffered extensive herpesvirus infection. Since skin infections among sportsmen represented a serious problem at that time various preventive measures including personal hygiene and environmental health programs were worked up. Such measures apparently subdued the outbreak because no similar epidemics of cutaneous herpes simplex have been reported lately.

III Herpesvirus infections of the fingers

The first histologic description of herpetic infection involving the eyelids of a nurse attending a child with eczema herpeticum was that of Juliusberg in 1898 (cit. by Lynch 1945). The earliest report of traumatic herpes occurring in the fingers — *herpes digitorum* — appears to be that of Adamson in 1909. He described four children with herpetic eruptions on the fingers (cit. by Ward and Clark 1961). Subsequently this form of herpetic infection was reported by the French authors Nicolau and Poincloux (1924), who isolated herpesvirus from vesicular lesions on the fingers of two patients.

Cases of digital herpes in nurses attending children with herpetic stomatitis of Kaposi's varicelliform eruptions have been reported by many authors (cit. by Simpson 1953). In 1956, Brain described herpetic lesions on the fingers of a pathologist and five nurses.

In 1959, Stern and associates presented a comprehensive study on the occurrence of herpetic nodular vesicles — *"herpetic whitlow"* — on the fingers of 54 nurses on the neurosurgical unit. Serologic studies revealed primary infection in about 90 percent of the cases. Herpetic efflorescences were localized predominantly on the index finger. In almost all cases the disease lasted for at least 2 weeks. At first the lesions were mistaken for a staphylococcal infection and were often treated surgically. Later, herpesvirus was isolated from vesicular fluid and traced to the tracheobronchial secretions of patients.

The view that herpetic infection of the fingers represents an occupational hazard for physicians, nurses and dentists has been amply confirmed (Ward and Clark 1961; Bart and Fisher 1965; Kanaar 1967; Brightman and Guggenheimer 1970; Wukelich 1972).

A small outbreak of herpetic whitlow totaling 4 patients within 10 days among nurses in a surgical intensive-care unit was recently reported by Hamory *et al.* (1975). The recommended gloving of both hands upon exposure to oropharyngeal secretions of patients seems logical but is excessive from an economic point of view (Orkin 1975).

The incubation period of primary herpetic infection involving fingers apears to be 3 to 7 days (Hambrick and Cox 1962; Kanaar 1967).

In 1971, Green and Levin reported an unusual case of primary herpetic infection in which the lesions progressed from the fingers to the oral cavity. This indicates that in cases of herpetic whitlow, herpesvirus may spread and cause lesions in other parts of the body.

Digital herpetic infection usually involves the thumb and index finger, and it is usually very painful. The infection is localized predominantly around the fingernails, and assumes a form that has been described as *herpetic paronychia* (Rosato *et al.* 1970; Brightman and Guggenheimer 1970). In the majority of the cases reported, herpetic infections of the fingers were associated with oral herpes (Nicolau and Poincloux 1924; Dodd *et al.* 1938; Slavin and Ferguson 1950; Ruiter 1950; Ward and Clark 1961; Hambrick and Cox 1962).

Autoinoculation of the herpesvirus in small children from the oral cavity to the fingers and vice versa has been noted by several authors (Burnet and Williams, 1939; Scott *et al.* 1952). Vivel *et al.* (1957), for instance, describe a case of a 4-year old child with herpetic stomatitis in whom direct inoculation of herpesvirus into the skin of the index finger occurred by sucking the finger ("Lutsch infektion"). Ten years later, Perol and Laufer (1967) reported the case of an adolescent in whom autoinoculation of the virus into the nail tissue occurred as a result of nail biting. That nail biting may be a significant factor in localizing the infection on the fingers has been emphasized by Muller and Herrmann (1970), who presented 2 cases of their own and 15 cases from the literature.

Herpetic infections of the fingers are an occupational hazard for medical and dental personnel who handle secretions from asymptomatic as well as symptomatic carriers (LaRossa and Hamilton 1971). Those who have never had a primary herpetic infection are at special risk. In the majority of the cases observed herpetic infection of the fingers occurred as a primary infection. Recurrent herpes of the fingers is unusual, although it has been noted in some instances.

Up to the present time it has not been determined which of the two types of herpesvirus causes infections of the fingers. According to Nahmias (1972), infections occurring above the waistline are caused by type 1, below the waist by type 2. Because of the multifunctional use of the fingers, herpetic whitlow may conceivably be caused by either of the two types.

Very often herpetic infections of the fingers are mistaken for pyoderma, bacterial paronychia, dermatitis, and herpes zoster. The differential diagnosis from subcutaneous bacterial infection is particularly important because surgical intervention may prolong the course of the disability.

Herpetic infection of the fingers has long been known as a clinical form of primary infection, but was recognized as an occupational hazard for medical and dental personnel only recently. Thus the differential diagnosis with some other conditions is of utmost importance.

IV Herpesvirus infection in burned patients

The susceptibility of burned patients to bacterial wound infection has been well documented. However topical and general prophylaxis with antibacterial agents has significantly reduced the frequency of these burn complications. Instead, viral burn-wound infections are recognized with increasing frequency.

Scott *et al.* (1952) were the first to report herpetic burn-wound infection in a 2-year-old girl who burned her finger on a cigarette. Her mother, who had a history of recurrent labial herpetic infection, "kissed it better." Several days later herpetic vesicular lesions developed on the child's hand and arm, from which HVH was isolated.

Foley *et al.* (1970) have published six cases of herpes simplex infection in patients with healing burns. Two of them died with a disseminated herpetic infection. On autopsy necrotizing hepatic and adrenal lesions similar to those described in neonatal herpetic infection were found, and all patients lacked neutralizing antibodies. Herpetic burn-wound infection is analogous to the extensive herpetic infection that occurs in eczematous children (see Chapter 8). The viral infection may have been primary but the possibility of a reactivated infection that resulted in extensive disease due to a post-traumatic immunologic defect cannot be excluded.

Nash and Foley (1970) found six cases of herpetic infection of the respiratory tract at autopsy during an outbreak of HVH infection in burned patients. In a review of past autopsy findings in their burned patients eight additional cases of histologically documented herpetic involvement of the middle and lower respiratory tract were found.

It would be interesting to have more virus isolations so as to know whether the etiologic agent in burn-wound superinfection was type 1 or type 2 HVH (*Brit. Med. J.* 1970).

The report of Foley *et al.* (1970) prompted Gallagher (1970) to describe the case of a 2-year-old girl who had typical herpesvirus eruptions on her palm and a history of burn-wound on the same hand. Local manifestations of the infection were small erosive lesions on the healing areas but particularly on the unburned areas of the skin. In the same issue of *The New England Journal of Medicine*, Torstenson *et al.* (1970) reported an additional example of a virus (vaccinia virus) infection in a burned child.

From these reports it is clear that extensively burned patients should be searched for infections with viruses. Superinfection with herpesvirus is a rare but not an impossible complication.

Chapter 13

HERPES HEPATITIS

Herpesvirus is the most protean of viruses in the wide variety of diseases it can cause.

Though hepatitis may be associated with various viruses, such as those of infectious and serum hepatitis (A and B), mononucleosis, yellow fever, and cytomegaloviruses, it had not until recently been reported with herpesvirus except in the neonatal period, when it occurs as a component of a widespread primary infection with the virus.

Tolentino and DeMatteis (1953) were the first to suspect herpesvirus as the causative agent of hepatitis in a 4-year-old child with primary herpetic infection. They found intranuclear inclusions in the liver tissue obtained by biopsy.

A few years later cases of herpetic hepatitis among infants and small children were reported from South Africa (McKenzie *et al.* 1959). There was an obvious association with malnutrition and measles. Febrile herpetic infection, usually stomatitis, was accompanied by enlargement of the liver, hypoglycemia, purpura, bleeding tendencies and a rise in serum aminotransferase indicating severe hepatitis. At necropsy, classical necrotizing lesions were usually present in the liver. The adrenals and other organs were also often affected.

The first case of herpes hepatitis in an adult was described by Flewett *et al.* (1969). They reported herpetic hepatitis in a pregnant woman, who survived. Liver biopsy confirmed the diagnosis of hepatitis, showing areas of necrosis and intranuclear inclusions characteristic of herpes. HVH was isolated from the mouth and from the liver tissue. Primary herpetic infection was confirmed by serologic tests. Electron microscopy showed herpesvirus-like particles in the nuclei of liver cells. The patient was delivered of a macerated fetus, 4 weeks after the onset of hepatitis. Unfortunately, virologic study was not carried out on the fetus.

Moglievska (1969) reports high herpetic antibody titer in the serum of a group of patients with hepatitis suggesting a possible association of this disease with HVH infection.

Diderholm et al. (1969) published a case of an elderly man who had bronchial asthma for many years and who died of generalized herpes infection associated with stomatitis. This was considered to be a rare instance of primary infection in an old patient. HVH was isolated from the liver. The hepatitis might have been due to the corticosteroid therapy. Administration of steroids probably favored the dissemination of HVH and eventual hepatic necrosis due to the infection in an adult with fulminant hepatitis reported by Francis et al. (1972).

Disseminated herpetic infection in the liver and adrenals has been described in adult patients suffering from extensive burns; in three such patients features of fulminant hepatic failure were manifested during life, though in two of these the diagnosis of HVH infection was not made until after death. The viral infection may have been primary but the possibility of reactivated infection was not excluded. Serological examination failed to demonstrate the presence of neutralizing antibodies to herpesvirus antigen before or after development of herpetic infection in another patient who died with disseminated lesions (Brit. Med. J. 1970).

An association of two viruses with the etiology of hepatitis is evidenced by the isolation of Coxsackie B5 and herpesvirus in fatal cases of hepatitis in siblings (Marks et al. 1969).

Goyette et al. (1974) describe a case similar to that reported by Flewett et al. (1969) of generalized herpes infection occurring in a pregnant woman. The overwhelming infection with HVH was acquired from the firstborn child, who had had herpetic gingivostomatitis in the preceding weeks. The diagnosis was not suspected until necropsy revealed an enlarged yellow-tan colored liver dotted with circular hemorrhagic rings. Histologic examination showed typical inclusion bodies and HVH was cultured from the liver and other organs.

Although Goyette et al. (1974) suggest that pregnancy infection is due to depressed immunological responses, the paucity of cases makes this suggestion difficult to accept (Brit. Med. J. 1973).

In all cases of fulminant hepatic failure the causal role of herpesvirus must be considered. Scrapings from any vesicles found on the body can be examined by optical microscopy for the typical inclusion bodies, which on electron microscopy can be seen to contain virus particles. Immunofluorescent staining is specific if liver biopsy is possible. All material obtained should also be cultured for the virus.

The decision to use antiviral drugs is difficult because IDU may be hepatotoxic and cytarabine may cause bone marrow depression (Dölle 1972; Brit. Med. J. 1974).

Chapter 14

ASSOCIATION OF ERYTHEMA EXUDATIVUM MULTIFORME WITH HERPES SIMPLEX

Urbach (1933) was the first to draw attention to erythema exudativum multiforme (EEM) occurring 7 to 10 days after an attack of herpes simplex. Forman and Whitwell (1934) were apparently unaware of Urbach's work when they reported 12 cases of EEM associated with herpes simplex. This association was that herpes precedes an attack of EEM or recurrent herpes commonly occurs in patients with EEM (Urbach 1937). Since that time their observations have been confirmed by a number of additional observations in the literature (Anderson 1945, Murray 1947, Rook 1947, Ustvedt 1948). The herpetic etiology of this syndrome was always established by clinical or serologic means or by inoculation on rabbit eye. A strain of herpesvirus has been isolated from the lung of a patient who died with an atypical pneumonia and EEM (Morgan and Finland 1949). In some studies attempts to isolate the virus were negative or the isolation revealed a virus-like agent but proof of herpes simplex was not conclusive (Anderson *et al.* 1949).

Evidence that the vesicular fluid from vulvar or cutaneous lesions contained herpesvirus has been obtained by inoculating the fluid into chorioallantoic membrane, where characteristic pocks were produced (Womack and Randall 1953, Foerster and Scott 1958).

Herpesvirus type 2 was isolated from skin lesions in a female with simultaneous genital herpes (McDonald and Feiwel 1970), and in a young man with recurrent erythema multiforme who was associated with culture-proven genital herpetic infection (Britz and Sibulkin 1975).

The significance of HVH in the etiology of erythema exudativum is very suggestive in the publication by Nasemann (1964) from the dermatologic clinic in Munich. In a retrospective analysis of 405 cases of patients with histories of EEM a preceding attack of herpes disease was confirmed in 15 percent and found to be very probable in another 17 percent. Thus a herpetic etiology seemed to be plausible in $15+17-32$ percent of the patients in this extensive clinical material.

Nasemann enlarged this study of herpetic etiology in a prospective follow-up of all patients with EEM in one year. Virologic and serologic findings confirmed HVH in 50 percent of these cases. Juretić et al. (1964) have reported a series of 29 cases in Yugoslavia. A herpetic etiology was established in 4 cases and was very probable in 2. This rate of incidence (20 percent) is lower than those given in previous publications.

Erythema exudativum multiforme is associated with primary as well as recurrent herpetic infections (Nasemann 1964, Juretić et al. 1964, Pandi 1964). The youth of the patients, the clinical picture, and the serologic increase of antibodies are indicative of primary herpetic disease.

Little has been reported about herpesvirus as a possible antigen. Söltz-Szötz (1963) reports a case in which erythema multiforme developed while the patient was receiving a herpesvirus vaccine for recurrent herpes simplex. Shelley (1967) reports a patient with recurrent postherpetic attacks of EEM. Intradermal tests with a formaldehyde-inactivated HVH antigen produced what appeared clinically and histologically to be erythema exudativum. This is taken as evidence that EEM can be due to a hypersensitivity to HVH. This was the first time that EEM had been provoked by an intradermal test. Such a skin test with herpes antigen could help to objectively distinguish postherpetic EEM from the other forms.

In a review of 122 cases of EEM, Ström (1969) found 8 in which the herpetic etiology was proved. He considered that there are strong reasons for regarding postherpetic EEM as a form of allergic reaction and not as herpetic sepsis with cutaneous manifestations.

Chapter 15

HERPESVIRUSES AND CARCINOMA

The several herpesviruses have recently been associated with tumors in various animal species (Goodheart 1970, Rabson 1972): the lymphoma of chickens called Marek's disease, the Lucke renal adenocarcinoma of frogs, ileocecal proliferative disease (possibly an adenocarcinoma) of hamsters, a leukemia of guinea pigs, a lymphoma of cottontail rabbits, and a lymphoma of monkeys.

The herpesviruses have been definitely linked causally to cancer in some species and therefore all herpesviruses are rendered suspect of the same capability.

In humans, herpesviruses have been associated with oncogenicity in the case of Epstein-Barr virus (EBV) in Burkitt's lymphoma and in nasopharyngeal carcinoma (Epstein *et al.* 1965; Henle *et al.* 1967, 1968, 1969; Ito *et al.* 1969; Goldman *et al.* 1971; Dean *et al.* 1973); perhaps also in sarcoidosis (Hirschaut *et al.* 1970).

Although anecdotal clinical accounts of cancer of the lip and mouth arising at sites of recurring herpes simplex lesions continue to be reported, there is no solid epidemiological or other evidence associating HSV I with tumor induction in man (Epstein 1965).

In the middle of the 19th century, Domenigo Rigoni-Stern, the farsighted chief physician of a Verona hospital, raised the issue of marriage in relation to risk of uterine cancers (Rotkin 1973). His conclusions from mortality records were that more uterine cancers are found in married than in unmarried women and that such cancers are rare among unmarried women and almost absent in certain orders of nuns.

The observation that cervical carcinoma essentially behaves like a venereally transmitted disease, more prevalent in women who have multiple sex partners and who begin heterosexual activity early in life, has led to the suspicion that herpesvirus type 2 might be its causative agent. Later work has shown that the incidence of cervical carcinoma is significantly higher among promiscuous women who have experienced early sexual activity. This observation suggested the possibility that cervical carcinoma may be caused by an agent that is venereally transmitted. Thus, trichomoniasis, syphilis and smegma bacillus were frequently implicated as possible oncogenic agents.

Within the last decade, there has been a surge of interest in the possible association of herpesvirus type 2 and carcinoma of the uterine cervix. Extensive work along this line has been conducted in three centers in the United States, namely: Atlanta (Naib, Nahmias, Josey), Houston (Rawls, Melnick), and Baltimore (Aurelian, Royston).

Naib et al. (1966) were the first to demonstrate a high frequency of cervical dysplasia (aplasia) in women with a history of genital herpes. In extensions of this work, Josey et al. (1968) and Naib et al. (1969) found that women with either carcinoma in situ or invasive disease had a genital herpes prevalence rate of 23.7 percent in contrast to controls who had a rate of only 2.7 percent.

Other workers have noted increased frequency of cervical anaplasia in women with genital herpes, ranging from 5.4 to 28 percent (An 1969; Ng et al. 1970b; Catalano and Johnson 1971; Naib et al. 1973). All reported studies demonstrate a positive correlation between cervical anaplasia and cytologically detected genital herpes.

With the possible exception of cytomegalovirus, genital herpetic infection is the most common infection of the uterine cervix.

Recent developments in viral cancerogenesis have shown that certain of the most common viruses of man may be oncogenic under appropriate circumstances and after an interval of dormancy (Josey et al. 1968, Rawls et al. 1968a, Nahmias et al. 1970d).

Epidemiologic characteristics and ecologic conditions demonstrate a marked similarity between women with genital herpes and those with cervical carcinoma (Rawls et al. 1968b). In general, there is a high degree of correlation between genital herpes and carcinoma of the cervix among Negro women of lower socioeconomic class, and among women with multiple sexual mates and early onset of sexual life. Cervical cancer is rare in children and nuns and it is less frequent among women of a higher socioeconomic status. The same applies to genital herpes (Josey et al. 1968).

The results of epidemiologic studies of cervical cancer suggest that women with the malignancy have attributes that would have placed them at a higher risk of acquiring venereal diseases than other women (Rotkin 1967; Martin 1967; Priden and Lilienfeld 1971).

Age distribution curves of the population with genital herpes and the population with cervical carcinoma are not identical but show a certain orderly correlation. Primary infection with type 2 HVH occurs most frequently between 17 and 25 years, whereas the median age for cervical dysplasia is about 26 years, for carcinoma in situ, 35 years, and for invasive carcinoma, 46 years. It seems evident that cancerous lesions are preceded by genital herpetic infection. The period from early adolescence to young adulthood seems to be the time of greatest risk of exposure or susceptibility to a sexually delivered cervical carcinogen (Naib *et al.* 1969).

The incidence of type 2 HVH antibodies is significantly higher among women with cervical carcinoma than among matched controls or women with other tumors (Aurelian *et al.* 1970; Rawls *et al.* 1969, 1970a; Naib *et al.* 1969; Royston and Aurelian 1970; Catalano and Johnson 1971; Plummer and Masterson 1971; Skinner *et al.* 1971). It has been stressed, however, that an association between antibodies to type 2 HVH and cervical neoplasia was found only in Negro women from lower socioeconomic groups in the United States but not in Caucasian women from higher socioeconomic groups in the United States and Europe (Rawls *et al.* 1969, 1970a; Sprecher-Goldberger *et al.* 1970; Centifanto *et al.* 1971). Antibodies to HVH type 2 show a typical variability with regard to population, race, age and socioeconomic status (Table 1).

Table 1. *The prevalence of HVH type 2 antibodies in women without carcinoma* (*Singer* 1971).

Population examined	Percentage with HVH type 2 antibodies
New Zealand, Caucasian women (mean age 42 years)	22
Baltimore, higher socioeconomic groups	41
Houston, prostitutes	54
Baltimore, lower socioeconomic groups	61
Baltimore, women over 45	71
Atlanta, women with history of genital herpes	91

Two basic methods have been used to assay antibodies to herpesvirus type 2: measurement of the kinetics of neutralization and measurement of total neutralizing activity. A summary of the results of studies in which the kinetics of neutralization was used is shown in Table 2.

Table 2. *Occurrence of antibodies to HSV type 2 in cervical cancer and controls (antibodies measured by kinetics of neutralization)*

Area	Race	Percentage of positive cancer cases	Percentage of positive controls	Reference
Houston	Negro	72	22	Rawls *et al.* (1969)
Baltimore	Negro	100	67	Royston and Aurelian (1970)
Brussells	White	83	33	Sprecher-Goldberger *et al.* (1970)
Copenhagen	White	85	47	Vestergard *et al.* (1972)
Chicago	White	48	18	Plummer and Masterson (1971)

The ratio of occurrences of herpetic antibodies in the cancer cases to occurrences in the controls is between 1.5 and 3.3.

A summary of reported studies in which antibodies were measured by determining end-point neutralization titers (micro-neutralization) is shown in Table 3. There was considerable variation in the percentage of women with cancer and of control women who were recorded with type 2 antibody activity (Kessler *et al.* 1974).

The incongruities in the results of the sero-epidemiologic studies may, in part, be ascribable to technical difficulties in assaying antibodies to HVH type 2. The antibody response to the specific antigens of type 2 virus may be diminished or absent when a type 2 virus infection occurs in an individual who has previously experienced a type 1 infection (Smith *et al.* 1972b).

From these and similar studies it is evident that there is a close association between the incidence of HVH type 2 antibodies and cervical carcinoma. According to some workers the rate of serologically positive findings increases progressively with the severity of lesions. This is shown in Table 4.

Table 3. *Occurrence of antibodies to HVH type 2 in cervical cancer and controls (antibodies measured by microneutralization test)*

Area	Race	Percentage of positive cancer cases	Percentage of positive controls	Reference
Atlanta	Negro	83	35	Nahmias *et al.* (1970a)
Uganda	Negro	93	72	Adam *et al.* (1972)
Houston	Negro	80	44	Rawls *et al.* (1973)
Houston	White	54	25	Rawls *et al.* (1973)
Virginia	White	52	23	Rawls *et al.* (1973)
Taiwan	Yellow	48	50	Rawls *et al.* (1973)
Colombia		37	35	Rawls *et al.* (1973)
Israel	White	38	27	Priden *et al.* 1971
New Zealand	White	31	23	Rawls *et al.* 1970a

Table 4. *Prevalence (percent) of HVH type 2 antibodies among women with preclinical and clinical cervical carcinoma (Nahmias et al. 1970a; Royston and Aurelian 1970; Rawls et al. 1969, 1970a; McDonald et al. 1974b).*

Type of lesion	Houston	Atlanta	Baltimore	Montreal
Dysplasia	24	56	95	40
Carcinoma in situ	35	70	100	40
Invasive carcinoma	78	83	100	35
Control groups	22	18—34	50—55	21—38

From all the data presented here, it is evident that there is a marked variation in the incidence of HVH type 2 antibodies among different groups of women. As shown, the incidence varies from 18 percent among women from higher socieconomic groups to 55 percent in Negro women from lower socioeconomic groups. The difference between the rates of preclinical lesions noted in the three studies may be due to differences in the serologic techniques used in these studies.

The work reported by Rawls et al. (1970a) and by Nahmias et al. (1971) suggests a progressive increase in the incidence of HVH type 2 antibodies from women with precancerous conditions to women with evident cancerous lesions.

It is well known that a precancerous condition does not necessarily lead to the development of invasive carcinoma. According to Rawls et al. (1970a), the incidence of dysplasias that differentiate into carcinoma seems to be identical with the incidence of dysplasias associated with the presence of HVH antibodies. Thus, it seems logical to conclude that the risk of developing invasive carcinoma is greater in women with dysplasia or carcinoma in situ and HVH type 2 antibodies than in women with such lesions but without antibodies.

Cells infected with herpesvirus type 1 or type 2 develop surface antigens that can be detected by immunofluorescence. In the series of Smith et al. (1972b) among women with cervical cancer the titers of antibodies detected by immunofluorescence as with antibodies detected by neutralization, were similar to those found in serum from selected control women. The surface fluorescence test provided no advantages over the microneutralization test in distinguishing women with cervical cancer from controls.

The results of a recent sero-epidemiological survey published by McDonald et al. (1974b) are not congruent with previously reported studies (Table 4).

Several explanations for different findings might be given and include the difficulty of detecting HSV-2 antibodies in indivuduals with prior HSV-1 infection. Another possibility is the variability in geographic strains of HSV and different causes of cervical cancer of which HSV may only be one (Nahmias et al. 1976).

Experimental work has shown that inoculation of HVH type 2 into hamsters results in the development of sarcoma (Nahmias et al. 1970d). Normal hamster embryo cells inoculated with HVH type 2 transformed into fibrosarcoma cells (Rapp and Duff 1972, 1973). On the basis of these findings herpesvirus has been included in the group of oncogenic viruses.

Evidence has been obtained for the *presence of HVH type 2 within tumor cells*. Thus, Aurelian et al. (1971, 1972) report the isolation of a herpesvirus from degenerated cervical tumor cells grown in vitro. On the basis of biologic and immunologic properties the virus was identified as HVH type 2. It appears that tumor cells harbor the viral genome in a repressed state and that exposure of the cells to high pH induces virus expression. By using the immuno-fluorescent technique, Frenkel *et al.* (1972) were able to demonstrate the presence of a DNA fragment of herpes virion in anaplastic cells of cervical carcinoma in vivo and in cell cultures. The presence of a fragment of DNA and not of the whole viral genome in tumor cells might perhaps explain why the virus failed to damage the infected host cells. Nevertheless, the presence of herpesvirus in neoplastic cells does not necessarily imply that the virus is responsible for the malignant transformation. On the other hand, it is difficult to suppose that there is no causal relation between them (Nahmias and Roizman 1973).

Three hypotheses have been advanced to account for the association of HVH type 2 and cervical carcinoma. First, it is possible that infection with HVH and cervical neoplasia are independent of each other but are both associated with sexual activity. Second, herpesvirus might be a secondary invader of neoplastic cells which are more susceptible to infection than normal cells. Third, the virus may attack cervical cells and act as an etiologic agent, either directly or as a cocarcinogen, in the induction of carcinoma (Royston and Aurelian 1970, Catalano and Johnson 1971).

In all populations thus far examined the greater neutralizing activity to HVH type 2 among patients than among control women appears to represent something more than a difference in sexual activity and a property associated with reproduction. The differences in antibody activity between women with cancer and control women do not appear to be due to dissimilarities between the groups in sexual promiscuity. Controls who are selected with similar attributes of sexual activity and reproduction-associated factors still have less antibody activity to the type 2 virus than the cancer patients.

The first *prospective studies* of the association between HVH type 2 infection and cervical carcinoma had control groups matched for age, race and socioeconomic and marital status. However, they were not matched for sexual activity (Nahmias and Roizman 1973; Rawls *et al.* 1973). Recent studies made use of two additional variables: age of onset of sexual activity and number of different sexual partners (Rotkin 1973). The data obtained from these studies also indicate a significant prevalence of HVH type 2 antibodies among women with cervical carcinoma. Thus, Rawls *et al.* (1973) found a rate of 43 percent in carcinoma patients compared to 17 percent in control groups. Royston and Aurelian (1970) reported that there is no association between cervical neoplasms and two other venereal diseases, syphilis and trichomonas infection.

Particular susceptibility of atypical cervical epithelium to HVH has been pointed out in several studies (Amstey 1973). The progressively higher rates of herpetic infection associated with increasing severity of neoplastic lesions suggest the possibility that HVH type 2 is a secondary invader of an altered cervical tissue (Rawls et al. 1969, 1970a).

This possibility is further borne out by a prospective study by Nahmias et al. (1973b) involving 871 women with herpes and 562 control women. They showed that the rate of cervical dysplasia was twofold greater, and that of carcinoma in situ eightfold higher in women with herpes than in the control group. The twofold-higher rate of carcinoma in situ was found in women in whom herpetic infection was established during pregnancy.

In the prospective study of Catalano and Johnson (1971) carcinoma in situ developed in HVH type 2 positive women at a rate four times higher than in control women. The data of this study lend support to the hypothesis that HVH type 2 may be the cause of cervical cancer rather than a secondary invader of neoplastic tissue.

From the results presented by Nahmias et al. (1973b) it appears that the rate of development of cervical anaplasia following a primary genital herpetic infection is not as high as the rate established in women whose infection was not identified as primary. It might be that recurrent HVH type 2 infection increases the opportunity for cell transformation by herpesvirus. The significance of recurrent infection obviously requires further study.

The availability of a tumor register in Sweden made it possible to determine the number of women in the herpes and control groups who developed cervical cancer in later years. A significantly higher frequency of neoplasma was observed in the herpes group, particularly in patients in whom genital herpes was diagnosed when they were 15—19 years old (Jeansson and Molin 1974 — cit. by Nahmias et al. 1976).

Although the association of HVH type 2 infection and cervical carcinoma seems to be very probable, there are still many gaps in our knowledge regarding the mechanism of the virus action. It is not known what is the nature of the urogenital-tract cells in which the virus is harbored, or when and how the virus multiplies. Also, there is no explanation of the low frequency of penile cancer as compared with that of cervical cancer, even though HVH infection also occurs commonly in males (Roizman and Frenkel 1973).

Martinez (1969) found eight patients with cervical carcinoma among the wives of 889 men with squamous cell carcinoma of the penis. He concluded that the two cancers might have HVH type 2 as a common etiological factor.

The similarities in the epidemiological patterns for genital HSV infection and cervical cancer provide one of the most difficult problems in establishing causality. An individual who acquires one venereally transmitted agent is likely to be exposed to other agents, either concurrently or at another time.

Nevertheless, recent studies identify women with HVH type 2 infection as a population at risk that requires careful Papanicolaou cervicovaginal screening for cervical neoplasia.

The data that have been presented clearly indicate that there is an association between HVH type 2 infection and cervical cancer, but the evidence for a causal relation is incomplete. Further confirmation should be obtained that viral antigen or the viral genome is present in anaplastic cells and cell lines derived from cervical carcinoma, that this virus can induce malignant transformation in human cells, and that cells transformed by this agent and cells derived from cervical malignancies contain closely related or identical tumor-specific antigens. The finding of a high frequency of antibodies to special well-characterized or type-specific HVH antigens in the serum of women with cervical cancer as compared to a well-controlled group of women without neoplasma must be confirmed (Nahmias *et al.* 1976).

The final proof of the association between genital herpes and cervical carcinoma must await further prospective studies involving groups of women who are in some way protected, as by immunization, from developing HVH type 2 infection. Such studies should determine whether the expected frequency of cervical carcinoma was reduced in the protected population. With regard to this, the development of a vaccine against HVH type 2 would be of interest (Poste *et al.* 1972; Nahmias and Roizman 1973). Even if HVH-2 can be shown to induce cervical cancer, the possibility of other causes, including other infectious agents, cannot be eliminated.

In a recent review Sabin (1975) expressed doubt about evidence that herpesviruses alone or in conjunction with some unknown factors are involved in any human cancer.

This chapter can be concluded with the recent citation from *British Medical Journal* (1976): "With steadily increasing evidence of a close link between the virus and cervical cancer the time may not be far off when firm diagnosis of HSV-2 infection warrants the more expensive fluorescent antibody test or even virus culture. Those women with a positive result could be kept under careful surveillance with frequent colposcopic and smear checks, for they seem to be at considerable risk."

Chapter 16

THERAPY OF HERPESVIRUS INFECTIONS

There have been numerous attempts to treat cutaneous herpesvirus infections either by various chemical agents or by immunologic and physical techniques. The chemical agent that has been most used is *5-iodo-2-deoxyuridine (IDU)*. In 1961, Calabresi *et al.* screened IDU for antitumor activity and noted that a greater inoculum of vaccinia virus was required to produce dermal lesions in rabbits receiving this compound. This finding suggested that IDU might be effective in certain DNA-virus infections. It interferes with incorporation of thymidine into viral DNA and produces an ineffective deceitful DNA molecule (Calabresi 1963). In other words, cells infected with herpesvirus use IDU in place of thymidine to replicate new virus and produce a faulty virus that is incapable of infecting other cells. It should be noted, however, that IDU interferes with the incorporation of thymidine into both host and viral DNA (Corbett *et al.* 1966).

However, experimental and clinical trials with IDU produced rather ambiguous results varying from excellent to completely negative. In the work of Corbett *et al.* (1969) the therapeutic efficacy of IDU was found to depend upon the times at which treatment was initiated and discontinued, the concentration of the drug and the solvent used. It appeared that IDU was ineffective if given within the first 2 hours following infection and then withdrawn. However, if the agent was left in situ or applied 4 hours or longer after virus inoculation, irreversible inhibition occurred. Apparently the agent must be present at the site of infection for a prolonged period of time in order to completely suppress the synthesis of new infectious virus.

The selection of an appropriate solvent that will prolong contact time of medication and promote percutaneous absorption also seems to be important for effective IDU treatment. Several solvent systems have been tested and polyvinyl alcohol found to

9

best fulfill the foregoing requirements. IDU appears to be most effective in a concentration of 0.1 percent. Greater concentrations were shown to be less effective, presumably because they alter the metabolic processes required for transport of the drug across the cell membrane (Corbett et al. 1966). Local application of IDU in herpetic keratitis has been successful (Kaufman 1962). The use of IDU to prevent experimentally induced herpetic infection in rabbits eye was unsuccessful (Juretić and Ribarić 1970).

Studies of the toxicity and urinary excretion of IDU revealed that significant blood levels are maintained for approximately 4 hours and that 5-iodo-uracil and iodide are excreted in the urine. The toxic effects of IDU seem to be related to its capacity to inhibit rapidly proliferating tissues. Toxic manifestations resulting from inhibited metabolism of these tissues include leukopenia, thrombocytopenia, stomatitis, alopecia, and nail ridging. Cholestatic jaundice may develop in patients treated by systemic use of IDU Dayan and Lewis 1969). These side effects of the agent have (been found to be related to dosage. Thus, they were found only occasionally in patients receiving less than 400 mg/kg, but were present in about two-thirds of patients given total doses of 400—600 mg/kg, and in all patients treated with over 600 mg/kg (Calabresi 1965).

The use of IDU in the treatment of cutaneous lesions resulting from herpesvirus has been reported in a number of papers. In 1962 Hall-Smith et al. reported rapid subjective amelioration of symptoms and healing of the lesions of cutaneous herpes within 2 to 5 days in 13 patients treated with IDU in the form of a 0.1 percent topical solution or a 0.5 percent ointment. On the other hand, Burnett and Katz (1963) failed to demonstrate any therapeutic benefit of IDU topically applied to 26 patients with herpesvirus infection of the skin. In their controlled double-blind trial IDU was applied in water soluble preparations at concentrations of 0.2, 2.0 and 10 percent. Similarly, Juel-Jensen and Mac Callum (1964) did not find any therapeutic effect of IDU applied to 27 patients presented with herpes simplex of the face. They report that the drug topically applied at a concentration of 0.5 percent in cream had no advantages over the placebo cream. Also relevant in this context is the finding of Ive (1964) that IDU had no significant effect on cutaneous herpesvirus infection.

However, in an extension of their work, MacCallum and Juel-Jensen (1966) tested the efficacy of a 5 percent solution of IDU in dimethyl sulfoxide. In 10 patients with recurrent herpesvirus of the face receiving this preparation they noted an average shortening of the expected duration of the lesions of 6.3 days (or 63 percent) and an average shortening of 2 days as compared with those receiving the solvent alone. This was the greatest reduction achieved thus far.

There is evidence that IDU is less effective against type 2 than type 1 herpesvirus (*JAMA* 1971).

Corbett *et al.* (1966) treated 111 patients for recurrent herpesvirus infections and reported that IDU-treated lesions showed a mean healing time of 5.7 days as compared with 12.5 days for untreated lesions. Similar results were obtained in herpes genitalis by Schofield (1964).

In an adult with severe primary herpesvirus stomatitis and pharyngitis with constitutional symptoms Alexander (1969) applied 0.1 percent IDU in spray to ulcers of the mouth and throat and achieved rapid relief of pain and probably a shortening of the course of the illness.

Nasemann and Braun-Falco (1970) treating 103 patients with ointment containing 0.2 percent IDU and 1.8 percent dimethylsulfoxide (DMSO), obtained results which suggested that the duration of the infection was shortened.

From all the data that have accumulated it appears that IDU hastens the healing of herpetic lesions but rarely eliminates the virus from the infected area. Published reports indicate that IDU suppresses virus replication in cell cultures without damaging the virus or the infected cells so that when the drug is withdrawn, virus replication recurs. Thus, the failure of IDU to eliminate herpesvirus from the skin might be similar to its effect in vitro (Tomlinson and MacCallum 1968).

Review of the literature concerning the treatment of severe herpesvirus infections with systemic IDU suggests that the side effects, although significant, are reversible and not fatal (Ashton *et al.* 1971). Several patients with severe infections have made good recoveries, which are probably ascribable to the drug (see relevant chapters). There have been many claims of success (Nolan *et al.* 1973) and failure with IDU in the treatment of herpesvirus encephalitis. Two placebo-controlled double blind studies have recently been reported from the United States in biopsy proved cases of HVH encephalitis, but IDU was abandoned because of therapeutic inactivity and inacceptable myelosuppression (Boston Interhospital Virus Study Group 1975; Editorial, *Lancet,* 1975).

Cytosine arabinoside (cytarabine or ara-C) is another agent effective against a number of DNA viruses in cell culture. Like IDU it is effective in treating herpetic keratitis in rabbits. The reported data indicate that cytarabine hinders the synthesis of viral DNA. (Falke *et al.* 1972; Fiala *et al.* 1972, 1974). In the experiments made by

9*

Underwood (1962) a combination of IDU and cytarabine was more efficient than either agent alone in treating herpesvirus keratitis in rabbits (Kaufman and Maloney 1963).

Juel-Jensen (1970) administered cytarabine to a patient with severe generalized herpesvirus infection. The benefit of the therapy was confirmed by a rapid regression of symptoms without any apparent toxic side effect from the drug.

The combined inoculation of cultures of human embryonic lung cells with herpesvirus type 2 and cytarabine produced a significant increase in the number of cells containing multiple chromatid and chromosome breaks. The possibility that chemical and viral mutagens act synergistically to produce chromosome abnormalities obviously warrants further investigation (O'Neill and Rapp 1971).

In the search for agents that might be effective against herpesvirus infection in man a number of other compounds have also been tested. It has been reported for some time that herpesvirus are sensitive to other inhibitors of viral DNA — 9-beta-D--arabinofuranosyladenine or *adenine arabinoside (ara-A)* — in cell cultures and in animals (Shardein and Sidwell 1968; Sidwell *et al.*, 1968). It has been reported that type 1 HVH was more sensitive to such inhibitors than was type 2. Person *et al.* (1970) demonstrated that the wide variation in sensitivity of HVH types 1 and 2 to antiviral agents (IDU and ara-A) results from differences in the cell culture system and passage history of the strain. When ara-A is given parenterally, it enters the cerebrospinal fluid readily. The results of a recent study, published by Ch'ien *et al.* (1975), suggest that ara-A, within its nontoxic dose range, may be efficacious in the treatment of neonatal HVH infection provided the drug is given early in the course of the disease.

At a San Francisco symposium on ara-A several participants reported that adenine arabinoside is at least as effective as IDU in the treatment of herpes simplex epithelial keratitis in humans. Ara-A (3 percent ointment) had a more rapid onset of action and was less toxic to the corneal epithelium that IDU (*JAMA* 1974).

In experimental HVH encephalitis in mice the fatal course was not altered by any dosage of cytosine arabinoside. On the other hand, treatment with adenine arabinoside resulted in long term survival of the majority of the infected animals (Sloan 1973; Griffith *et al.* 1975).

Azauridine (6-azauricil ribonucleoside) inhibits a variety of RNA and DNA viruses in culture. Inhibition of HVH replication has been reported by some authors (Falke and Rada 1970; Prusoff and Goz 1973). Azauridine was effective in the therapy of

HVH infection of the eye in rabbits and man. The inhibition of viral replication was in correlation with the activity of uridine kinase. Of potential importance is the observation that the simultaneous administration of 6-azauridine and a cell-free extract containing uridine kinase to infected cells in culture produced a marked increase in viral inhibition (Rada and Altanerova 1970; Rada and Hanušovskà 1970).

Dym and Becker (1969) assessed the efficacy of *p-fluoro-phenylalanine* (FPA), an inhibitor of RNA and DNA viruses. With a test system involving administration of FPA to herpesvirus-infected cultured cells they achieved inhibition of virus synthesis. However, low doses of FPA produced only a partial inhibitory effect.

Effective chemotherapy for virus infections is a challenge to biochemical ingenuity, since the complexity of the union between host and virus makes it difficult to inhibit the multiplication of the virus without at the same time damaging host cells (*Brit. Med. J.* 1974).

In a series of experiments, Underwood (1970) tested 4 — 2- -*nitro-1-(p-tolylthio) ethyl-acetanilide* or compound U-3243. The compound was active against experimental herpesvirus infection in rabbits but showed minimal activity against the virus in cultured cells and was no more effective than placebo when tested topically in man.

Krueger and Mayer (1970) undertook experiments with *tilorone hydrochloride*, a substance active against some RNA and DNA viruses. They noted a significant reduction in severity of herpesvirus infection in mice treated orally with tilorone, especially if treatment was initiated at least 24 hours prior to virus inoculation and continued daily for 7 days.

In a series of in vitro studies, Falke and Kahl (1971) assessed the effect of *compound 48/80*, a histamineliberating substance, on giant cell formation induced by HVH in cultured rabbit kidney cells. They showed that this agent inhibits the penetration of the virus into cells and that the phase of penetration sensitive to it begins immediately after infection and lasts for about 30 minutes. The penetration was not inhibited, however, when compound 48/80 was administered later than 30 minutes after infection and the synthesis of virus particles proceeded normally. Nevertheless, the compound inhibited the formation of giant cells in herpesvirus infected cultures even when giant cell formation had already started.

Okada and Kim (1972) examined the effect of *concanavalin A* on several viruses including herpesvirus. After treatment with the preparation, herpesvirus became noninfectious. The effect of concanavalin A was reversed by washing the virus with methyl-manoside, a specific inhibitor of concanavalin A. This finding suggested to the authors that like some other enveloped viruses, herpesvirus has receptors for concanavalin A on its surface. Concanavalin A binds with these receptors and converts the virus to the non infectious state.

The use of sugar analogs may offer a new approach to the treatment of herpesvirus infections. The sugar analog *2-deoxy--D-glucose* was effective in preventing or reducing the severity of herpetic keratitis in rabbits (Ray *et al.* 1974).

The antibiotics *rifamycin* and *distamycin A* have been tried in local therapy of cutaneous herpes, but the results were indefinite (Netter *et al.* 1972; Verini *et al.* 1972; Pascheta 1972).

Suppression of herpes simplex virus infection in an animal experiment by *phosphonoacetic acid* is reported by Shipkowitz *et al.* (1973) and Mao *et al.* (1975).

Some of the most exciting recent experimental work has involved the use of *interferon* and *interferon inducers* in the treatment of herpesvirus infection (Field *et al.* 1967). Hamilton *et al.* (1969) reported that synthetic double-stranded ribonucleic acids which induce interferon production protect against herpesvirus-induced cytopathogenicity in cell cultures, systemic herpesvirus infection in mice and herpetic keratoconjunctivitis in rabbits. They showed that polyribouridylic acid (poly-rA:rU) and polyribocytidylic acid (poly--rI:rC) reduced mortality in mice infected with HVH even when the treatment was started 24 hours after virus inoculation. In addition, they observed that both poly-rA:rU and poly-rI:rC prolonged the survival of infected mice even when administered 48 hours after virus inoculation. This finding is of particular importance since it is the first example of an antiviral agent that is efficient when given after virus infection (Catalano 1969).

Catalano and Baron (1970) administered poly-rI:rC to mice intracerebrally inoculated with herpesvirus and encephalomyocarditis virus (EMCV) and noted a significant delay in mortality and increased survival. However, the agent was found to be more effective against EMCV than against herpesvirus when increasing doses of the virus were inoculated.

Ikić *et al.* (1971) reported on the use of interferon in human herpesvirus infections. Patients with either labial or recurrent genital herpes were treated with interferon ointment (4 000 units of interferon per gram). The lesions treated within 48 hours of eruption regressed more rapidly than untreated lesions. The accompanying subjective symptoms disappeared after 3 to 5 days and in the majority of patients treated with interferon the remission lasted longer.

No beneficial effect to the infant could be noted from the intrathecal administration of interferon in neonatal herpes as used by De Clercq *et al.* (1975).

In addition to the use of chemotherapy in the prophylaxis and treatment of herpesvirus infections there have been several attempts to induce resistance by other techniques such as *immunization*. Thus, it has been reported that topical immunization of the rabbit conjunctiva and cornea with heat inactivated herpes virus conferred partial protection when sensitized animals were challenged with live herpesvirus. Topical immunization of rabbits resulted in the appearance of IgA specific antibodies and interferon in the tears from both eyes (Centifanto *et al.* 1970).

Bolgert and Tintoin (1965) successfully applied ultraviolet inactivated herpesvirus to 7 boys presented with severe gingivostomatitis. They reported that two consecutive subcutaneous injections of the inactivated vaccine resulted in rapid disappearance of herpetic lesions and malaise.

Many authors have attempted to prevent herpetic recurrences with *antiherpetic vaccine,* but the results were indefiinite (Lazar 1956; Henocq 1972; Vukas and Kon 1966; Pollikoff 1970; Santoianni 1966).

Another attempt to prevent recurrent herpesvirus infection involved *autoinoculation*. Fluid from a fresh herpetic vesicle was aspirated and inoculated by scarification or intradermal injection into another area of the body. It was noted, however, that autoinoculation may result in the induction of new foci of recurrent herpes (Goldman 1961).

Neff and Lane (1970) report data on 9 adult patients with hematologic malignancies in whom vaccinia necrosum occurred following *smallpox vaccination* as a therapeutic means for chronic herpetic ulcer. They rightly emphasize the hazards of smallpox vaccination as a treatment for recurrent HVH infection.

Nahmias *et al.* (1969d) tested the effect of *antithymocyte serum* on herpesvirus infections in mice. The results of their work indicate that rabbit antithymocyte serum increased mortality in mice intragenitally inoculated with herpesvirus but reduced or delayed mortality in intracerebrally infected animals.

Finally, a few words may be said regarding *physical treatment*. In 1970, Krashen used *cryotherapy* in an effort to eliminate herpesvirus from the mouth. He reported that recovery occurred within 24 to 48 hours when cryotherapy was applied within 3 days of the appearance of vesicles. In all but 2 of his 127 patients thus treated a single treatment was sufficient to stop formation of vesicles.

The immediate relief of pain and quick healing in some cases of herpes genitalis and herpes labialis with the local application of *ether* were reported almost concurrently from India by Pasricha *et al.* (1973) and from the United States by Nuget and Chou (1973): A controlled trial is necessary to substantiate these findings.

Wallis and Melnick (1965) have reviewed the dynamics of *photooxidation* of viruses and suggested that treatment of herpetic lesions with heterocyclic dyes followed by exposure to light might be clinically beneficial. Some recent studies have produced evidence that herpesvirus lesions respond to this unlikely sounding treatment (*JAMA* 1971; Felber 1971; Friedrich 1973). A controlled trial using neutral red gave some success (Felber *et al.* 1973). In these studies herpes genitalis due to type 2 virus appeared to be more sensitive to photoinactivation than that due to type 1 virus (Kaufman *et al.* 1973b).

Photodynamic inactivation was most effective with dyes such as neutral red, proflavine, toluidine blue, and acridine orange. The dye gets incorporated into the virus during the process of its replication. At this stage the virus becomes hypersensitive to light and can be inactivated by subsequent brief exposure to ordinary fluorescent light.

Methylene blue, a phenothiazine derivative, has been shown to be viricidally active toward herpesvirus hominis in the presence of light both in vitro and in vivo. Recently, a controlled study with local application of 0.1 percent methylene blue solution demonstrated therapeutic effectiveness in eczema herpeticum (Chang and Weinstein 1975; Chang 1975).

Recent double blind studies, reported by Myers *et al.* (1975) indicate that the neutral-red and light treatment of recurrent cutaneous and mucocutaneous lesions caused by herpes genitalis was not better than the placebo and light treatment.

The results of Rapp *et al.* (1973) indicate that HVH retains the capability to transform mammalian cells after photodynamic inactivation of infectivity.

Photodynamic inactivation of herpesvirus represents a new form of therapy which needs additional investigations and controlled trials (*Brit. Med. J.* 1974).

BIBLIOGRAPHY

Abadzhyan, G. A.: "Results subsequent to interferon treatment of patients with herpetic keratitis" *Vestn. Oftalmol.* 1 72, 74, 1968.

Abadzhyan, G. A., Balezina, T. I., Korabelnikova, N. I.: "Comparative evolution of the therapeutic efficacy of interferon preparations in herpetic keratitis" *Vestn. Oftalmol.* 2, 48, 1971.

Adam, E., Sharma, S. D., Zeigler, O., Iwamoto, K., Melnick, J. L., Lewy, A. H., Rawls, W. E.: "Seroepidemiologic studies of herpesvirus type 2 and carcinoma of the cervix. II, Uganda" *J. Nat. Cancer Inst.* 48, 65, 1972.

Adams, J. H., Jennett, W. B.: "Acute necrotizing encephalitis: a problem in diagnosis" *J. Neurol. Neurosurg. Psychiatry* 30, 248, 1967.

Adour, K. K., Bell, D. N., Hilsinger, R. L.: "Herpes simplex virus in idiopathic facial paralysis (Bell palsy)" *JAMA* 233, 527, 1975.

Afzelius-Alm, L.: "Aseptic (nonbacterial) encephalomeningitides in Gothenburg, 1932—1950. Clinical and experimental investigation with special reference to the viruses of herpes, influenza, mumps and lymphocytic choriomeningitis" *Acta Med. Scand. Suppl.* 140, 1, 1951.

Alexander, J. G.: "The use of idoxuridine in the treatment of severe acute primary herpes simplex stomatitis and pharyngitis in adults" *Brit. J. Clin. Pract.* 23, 36, 1969.

Alford, C. A., Foft, J. W., Blankenship, W. J.: "Subclinical central nervous system disease of neonates: a prospective study of infants born with increased levels of IgM" *J. Pediatr.* 75, 1167, 1969.

Allen, J. C., Watters, G., O'Gorman, A. M., Patriquin, H., Meloff, K., Middleton, P., Armstrong, D.: "Herpes virus type 2 encephalitis in two neonates from the same household" *J. Pediatr.* 89, 6, 949, 1976.

Allison, A. C.: "Immunity and immunopathology in virus infections" *Ann. Inst. Pasteur 123*, 585, 1972.

Altshuler, G.: "Pathogenesis of congenital herpesvirus infection" *Am. J. Dis. Child, 127*, 427, 1974.

Amin, P. H.: "Radiological findings in herpes simplex encephalitis," *Brit. J. Radiol.* 45, 652, 1972.

Amman, A., cit., by Cavara and Bietti, (1952): *Le manifestazioni occulari dell' infezione erpetica* (Licino Cappelli, Bologna, 1946).

138

Amstey, M. S.: "Management of pregnancy complicated by genital herpes virus infection" *Am. J. Obstet. Gynecol.* 37, 515 1970.

Amstey, M. S.: "Herpesvirus cervitis and cervical neoplasia" *Cancer* 32, 1321 1973.

Amstey, M. S., Balduzzi, P. C.: "Genital herpesvirus (type 2) strain differences" *Am. J. Obstet. Gynecol.* 108, 188, 1970.

An, S. H.: "Herpesvirus infection detected on routine gynecologic cell specimens" *Acta Cytol.* 13, 354, 1969.

Anderson, J. A., Bolin, V., Sutow, W. W., Kito, W.: "Virus as possible etiologic agent of erythema exudativum multiforme, bullous type" *Arch. Dermatol. Syph.* 59/3, 251, 1949.

Anderson, K.: "Pathogenesis of herpes simplex virus infection in chick embryos" *Am. J. Pathol.* 16, 136, 1940.

Anderson, N. P.: "Erythema multiforme: its relationship to herpes simplex" *Arch. Dermatol. Syph.* 51, 10, 1945.

Anderson, S. G., Hamilton, J.: "The epidemiology of primary herpes simplex" *Med. J. Austral.* 308, 1949.

Andrews, C. H., Carmichael, E. A.: "Presence of antibodies to herpesvirus in postencephalitis and other human sera" *Lancet 1*, 857, 1930.

Armengaud, M., Baylet, R. J., Cemain, R., Quexuonum, C., Guerin, M., Schleup, R.: "Note preliminaire à l'etude de la primoinfection herpetique de l'enfant africain (à propos de 244 observations)" *Bull. Soc. Med. Afr. Noire Lang. Fr.* 8, 358, 1963.

Armstrong, C.: "Herpes simplex virus recovered from the spinal fluid of a suspected case of lymphocytic choriomeningitis" *Public. Health. Rep.* 58, 16, 1943.

Ashton, H., Frenk, E., Stevenson, C. J.: "Herpes simplex virus infection and idoxuridine" *Brit. J. Dermatol.* 84, 496, 1971.

Aurelian, L.: "Possible role of herpes virus hominis type 2 in human cervical cancer" *Pediatr. Proc.* 31, 1651, 1972.

Aurelian, L., Roizman, B.: "Abortive infection of canine cells by herpes simplex virus. II, Alternative suppression of synthesis of interferon and viral constituents" *J. Mol. Biol.* 2, 539, 1965.

Aurelian, L., Royston, I., Hugh, J. D.: "Antibody to genital herpes simplex virus: association with cervical atypia and carcinoma in situ" *J. Natl. Cancer Inst.* 45, 455, 1970.

Aurelian, L., Strandberg, J. D., Melendez, L. V, Johnson, L. A.: "Herpesvirus type 2 isolated from cervical tumor cells grown in tissue culture" *Science 174*, 704, 1971.

Bach, C. H., Schaefer, P., Babinet, B.: "Primoinfection herpetique benigne chez un nouveau-né" — *Ann. Pediatr.* (Sem. Hop. Paris) 42, 1, 57, 1966.

Bahrani, M., Boxerbaum, B., Gilger, A.: "Generalized herpes simplex and hypoadrenocorticism" *Am. J. Dis. Child.* 11, 437, 1966.

Balfour, H. H., Loken, M. K., Blaw, M. E.: "Brain scan in a patient with herpes simplex encephalitis" *J. Pediatr.* 71, 405, 1967.

Barile, M. F., Blumberg, J. M., Kraul, C. W., Yagauchi, R.: "Penile lesions among U. S. armed forces personnel in Japan" *Arch. Dermatol.* 86, 273, 1962.

Baringer, J. R.: "Recovery of herpes simplex virus from human sacral ganglions" *New Eng. J. Med. 291*, 828, 1974.

Baringer, J. R.: "Herpes simplex virus in sensory ganglions" *New Eng. J. Med.* *292*, 51, 1975.

Baringer, J. R., Swoveland, P.: "Recovery of herpes simplex virus from human trigeminal ganglions" *New Eng. J. Med. 288*, 648, 1973.

Baron, A., Le Bourhis, S., Gouray, N.: "Action des corticosteroides sur les lesions herpetiques de la cornee" *Bull. Hem. Soc. Ophthalmol. Fr. 72*, 647, 1959.

Barrow, G. I.: "The herpes simplex virus in infantile eczema" *Brit. Med. J. 2*, 482, 1954.

Bart, J. B., Fisher, I.: "Primary herpes simplex infection of the hard: report of case" *J. Am. Dent. Assoc. 71*, 74, 1965.

Bastian, F. O., Rabson, A. S., Yes, C. L., Tralka, T. S.: "Herpesvirus hominis: isolation from human trigeminal ganglion" *Science 178*, 306, 1972.

Battignani, A.: "Congiuntivite da virus erpetico in neonato" *Boll. Oculist. 13*, 1217, 1934.

Bean, S. F., Fusaro, R. M.: "Atypical cutaneous herpes simplex infection associated with acute myelogenous leukemia" *Acta Derm. Ven. 149*, 94, 1969.

Becker, W.: "The epidemiology of herpesvirus infection in three racial communities in Cape Town" *S. Afr. Med. J. 40*, 109, 1966.

Becker, W., Naude, T., Kipps, A., McKenzie, D.: "Virus studies in disseminated herpes simplex infections" *S. Afr. Med. J. 37*, 74, 1963.

Becker, W. B., Kipps, A., McKenzie, D.: "Disseminated herpes simplex virus infection" *Am. J. Dis. Child.* 115, 8, 1968.

Behrman, S., Knight, G.: "Herpes simplex associated trigeminal neuralgia" *Neurology 4*, 525, 1954.

Beilby, J. O., Cameron, C. H., Catterall, R. D., Davison, D.: "Herpesvirus hominis infection of the cervix associated with gonorrhoea" *Lancet 1*, 1065, 1968.

Bellanti, J. A., Guin, G. H., Grassi, R. M., Olson, L. C.: "Herpes simplex encephalitis: brain biopsy and treatment with 5-iodo-2-deoxyuridine" *J. Pediatr. 72*, 266, 1968.

Bellanti, J. A., Catalano, I. W., Chambers, R. W.: "Herpes simplex encephalitis: virologic and serologic study of a patient treated with an interferon inducer" *J. Pediatr. 78*, 136, 1971.

Belošević-Vidić, D., Hirtzler, R.: "Generalizirani herpes simplex poslije morbila" (Generalised herpes simplex after measles) *Achriv ZMD* 12, 309, 1968.

Berg, J. W.: "Esophageal herpes: a complication of cancer therapy" *Cancer 8*, 731, 1955.

Berkovich, S., Ressel, M.: "Neonatal herpes keratitis" *J. Pediatr. 69*, 652, 1966.

Bernstein, M. T., Stewart, J. A.: "Method for typing antisera to herpesvirus hominis by indirect hemagglutination inhibition" *Appl. Microbiol. 21*, 680, 1971.

Biegeleisen, J. Z., Scott, L. V.: "Transplacental infection of fetuses of rabbits. with herpes simplex virus" *Proc. Soc. Exp. Biol. Med.* 95, 411, 1958.

Bird, T., Gardner, P. S.: "Disseminated herpes simplex in the newborn" *Brit. Med. J. 2*, 992, 1959.

Bird, T., Ennis, J. E., Wort, A. J., Gardner, P. S.: "Disseminated herpes simplex in newborn infants" *J. Clin. Pathol. 16*, 423, 1963.

Black, W. C.: "The etiology of acute infectious gingivostomatitis" *J. Pediatr.* *20*, 145, 1942.

Blackweed, W., Dudgeon, J. A., Newns, G. H., Phillips, B. M.: "Case of encephalitis due to herpes simplex" *Brit. Med. J. 1*, 1519, 1966.

Blagojević, M., Ilić, R.: "Savremena shvatanja u liječenju herpetičkih keratitisa" (Modern concepts in the management of herpetic keratitis) — *Acta Ophthalmol. Iug. 2*, 159, 1964.

Blank, H., Rake, G. W.: *Viral and Rickettsial Diseases of the Skin, Eye and Mucous Membranes of Man* (Little/Brown, Boston, 1954).

Bligh, A. S., Weaver, C. M., Wells, C. E. C.: "Isotope encephalography in the management of acute herpes virus encephalitis" *J. Neurol. Neurosurg. Psychiatry. 35*, 569, 1972.

Bobo, C. B., Antine, B., Manos, J. P.: "Neonatal herpes simplex infection limited to the cornea" *Arch. Ophthalmol. 84*, 697, 1970.

Bolgert, M. M., Tintoin, J. F.: "Un cas de gingivo-stomatite herpètique de primo-infection. Efficacité rapide du vaccin antiherpètique" *Bull. Soc. Franc. Derm. Syph. 72*, 11, 1965.

Bonamour, G.: *Ophtalmologie Clinique* (Doin-Deren, Paris, 1969), Vol. 1.

Booth, C. B., Okazaki, H., Gaulin, J. C.: "Acute inclusion encephalitis of herpes simplex type" *Neurology, 11*, 619, 1961.

Boston Interhospital Virus Study Group: "Failure of high dose of 5-ido-2-deoxyuridine in the therapy of herpes encephalitis" *New Eng. J. Med. 292*, 12, 599, 1975.

Bouè, A., Loffredo, V.: "Avortement causé par le virus de l'herpès" *Presse Med. 78*, 103, 1970.

Brain, R. T.: "The clinical vagaries of the herpes virus" — *Brit. Med. J. 1*, 1061, 1956.

Brain, R. T., Pugh, R. C. B., Dudgeon, J. A.: "Adrenal necrosis in generalised herpes simplex" *Arch. Dis. Child. 32*, 120, 1957.

Breeden, C. J., Hall, T. C., Tyler, H. R.: "Herpes simplex encephalitis treated with systemic 5-iodo-2-deoxyuridine" *Ann. Med. Interne 65*, 1050, 1966.

Brier, A. M., Snyderman, R., Mergenhagenm, S. E., Notkins, A. L.: "Inflammation and herpes simplex virus: release of a chemotaxis-generating factor from infected cells" *Science 170*, 1104, 1970.

Brier, A. M., Wohlenberg, C., Rosenthal J., Mage, M., Notkins, A. L.: "Inhibition or enhancement of immunological injury of virus infected cells" *Proc. Natl. Acad. Sci. USA 68*, 3073, 1971.

Brightman, V. J., Guggenheimer, J. G.: "Herpetic paronychia: primary infection of the fingers with herpes simplex virus" *J. Am. Diet. Assoc. 80*, 112, 1970.

Brit. Med. J. 2204, 1969: Leading article: "Herpes hepatitis."

Brit. Med. J. 618, 1970: Leading article: "Herpesvirus infection in burned patients."

Brit. Med. J. 1, 418, 1971. Leading article: "Herpes virus and psychiatric disorders."

Brit. Med. J. 1, 248, 1973. Leading article: "Herpes hepatitis in adults."

Brit. Med. J. 484, 1974. Leading article: "Hepatitis and herpes virus."

Brit. Med. J. 1, 671, 1976: Leading article: "Herpesvirus and cancer of uterine cervix."

Britz, M., Sibulkin, D.: "Recurrent erythema multiforme and herpes genitalis (type 2)" *JAMA 233*, 7, 812, 1975.

Brody, J., Seven, J. L., Hensen, T. E: "Virus antibody titers in multiple sclerosis patients, siblings and controls" *JAMA 216*, 9, 1441, 1971.

Brown, R. M.: "A Quantitative Study of the Inhibition of Herpes Simplex Virus by Interferon" thesis University of Texas, Austin, 1966 cit. by Kaplan, A. S. in (S. Gard, C. Hallauer and K. F. Meyer, eds.), *Herpes, Simplex and Pseudorabies Viruses* (Springer, New York, 1969), p. 78.

Brown, W., Ishizaka, M., Yayima, Y., Webb, D., Winchurch, R.: in (R. Beers and W. Brown, eds.,) *Biological effects of Polynucleotides* (Springer, New York, 1971), p. 26.

Brunell, P. A., Dodd, K.: "Isolation of herpes virus hominis from the cerebrospinal fluid of a child with bacterial meningitis and gingivostomatitis" *J. Pediatr.* 65, 63, 1964.

Buckley, T. F., MacCallum, F. O.: "Herpes simplex virus encephalitis treated with idoxuridine" *Brit. Med. J.* 2, 419, 1967.

Buddingh, G. I., Schrum, D. I., Lanier, J. C., Guidry, D. J.: "Studies of natural history of herpes simplex infection" *Pediatrics 11*, 595, 1953.

Burnet, F. M., I ush, D.: "Herpes simplex. Studies on the antibody content of human sera" *J. Pathol. Bacteriol.* 48, 275, 1939.

Burnet, F. M., Williams, S. W.: "Herpes simplex: a new point of view" *Med. J. Austral.* 26, 637, 1939.

Burnett, Y. W., Katz, S. L.: "Study of the use of 5-iodo-2-deoxyuridine in cutaneous herpes simplex" *J. Invest. Dermatol.* 40, 7, 1963.

Calabresi, P.: "Current status of clinical investigation with 6-azauridine, 5--iodo-2-deoxyuridine and related derivatives" *Cancer Res*, 23, 1260, 1963.

Calabresi, P.: "Clinical studies with systemic administration of antimetabolites of pyrimidine nucleosides in viral infections" *Ann. N. Y. Acad. Sci. 130*, 192, 1965.

Calabresi, P., Cardoso, S. S., Finch, S. C., Kligerman, M. M., Von Kesen, C. F., Chu, M. Y., Welch, A. A. D.: "Initial clinical studies with 5-iodo--2-deoxyuridine" *Cancer Res.* 21, 550, 9, 1961.

Caldwell, J. E., Porter, D. D.: "Herpetic pneumonia in alcoholic hepatitis" *JAMA 217*, 12, 1703, 1971.

Campinchi, M. R., Deniz-Lasalle, J.: "Raport de l'immunologie au diagnostic de l'herpès oculaire (étude de serum), de l'humeur aquese et des larmes" *Bull. Soc. Ophtalmol. Fr.* 67, 856, 1967.

Cantell, K., Tommila, V.: "Effect of interferon on experimental vaccinia and herpes simplex virus infections in rabbits' eyes" *Lancet* 2, 682, 1960.

Cappel, R., Klastersky, J.: "L'infection herpètique du systeme nerveux central. Diagnostic et traitement" *Nouv. Presse Med.* 1, 2395, 1972.

Carroll, J. M., Martola, E. L., Laibson, P. R., Dohlman, T. C. H.: "The recurrence of herpetic keratitis following idoxuridine therapy" *Am. J. Ophthalmol.* 63, 103, 1967.

Carton, C. A., Kilbourne, E. D.: "Activation of latent herpes simplex by trigeminal sensory-root section" *New Eng. J. Med.* 246, 172, 1952.

Casazza, A. R., Duvall, C. P., Carbone, P. P.: "Infection in lymphoma: histology, treatment and duration in relation to incidence and survival" *JAMA 197*, 710, 1966.

Castleman, B.: "Case records of the Massachusetts General Hospital, Case 61" *New Eng. J. Med. 271*, 1313, 1964.

Catalano, L.: "Poly I-poly C treatment of herpes (discussion)" *J. Pediatr.* 75, 1202, 1969.

Catalano, L. W.: "Herpesvirus hominis antibody in multiple sclerosis and amyotrophic lateral sclerosis" *Neurol.* 22, 475, 1972.

142

Catalano, L. W., Baron, S.: "Protection against herpes virus and encephalomyocarditis virus encephalitis with a double stranded RNA inducer of interferon" *Proc. Soc. Exp. Biol. Med. 133*, 684, 1970.

Catalano, L. W., Johnson, L. D.: "Herpesvirus antibody and carcinoma in situ of the cervix" *JAMA 217*, 447, 1971.

Catalano, L. W., Safley, G. H., Museles, M., Jarzynski, D. J. I "Disseminated herpesvirus infection in a newborn infant" *J. Pediatr. 79*, 3, 393, 1971.

Cavara, V., Bietti, G. B.: "Le manifestazioni oculari delle malattie da virus e da rickettisie" Relaz. al *XXXIX Congr. Soc. Oftal. Ital.* (Torino, 1952).

Cederqvist, L., Eliasson, G., Lindell, L., Stromby, K.: "Nuclear inclusion bodies in vaginal smears from patients with vaginal discharge" *Acta Obstet. Gynecol. Scand. 49*, 13, 1970.

Centifanto, Y. M., Kaufman, H. E.: "Secretory immunoglobulin A and herpes keratitis" *Infect. Immun. 2*, 788, 1970.

Centifanto, Y. M., Little, J. M., Kaufman, H. E.: "The relationship between virus chemotherapy, secretory antibody formation and recurrent herpetic disease" *Ann. N. Y. Acad. Sci 173*, 649, 1970.

Centifanto, Y. M., Mildebrandt, R. J., Held, B., Kaufman, H. E.: "Relationship of herpes simplex genitalis infection and carcinoma of the cervix: population studies" *Am. J. Obstet. Gynecol. 110*, 690, 1971.

Centifanto, Y. M., Drylie, D. M., Deardourff, S. L., Kaufman, H. E.: "Herpes type 2 in the male genitourinary tract" *Science 178*, 318, 1972.

Cesario, T. C., Poland, J. D., Wulff, H.: "Six years experience with herpes simplex virus in a children's home" *Am. J. Epidemiol. 90*, 416, 1969.

Chandler, J. W., Heine, E. R., and Weiser, R. S., in *Proceedings of the fourth Annual Leukocyte Culture Conference* (Appleton-Century-Crofts, New York, 1971), p. 227.

Chang, T. W.: "Methylene blue for eczema herpeticum" *JAMA 233*, 9, 987, 1975.

Chang, T. W., Solomon, P., Weinstein, L.: "Generalized fatal herpes simplex in a newborn infant. Demonstration of viruria" *J. Pediatr. 68*, 473, 1966.

Chang, T. W., Weinstein, L.: "Eczema herpeticum: treatment with methylene blue and light" *Arch. Dermatol. 111*, 1174, 1975.

Charnock, E. L., Cramblett, H. C.: "5-Iodo-2-deoxyuridine in neonatal herpesvirus hominis encephalitis" *J. Pediatr. 76*, 3, 459, 1970.

Ch'ien, L. T., Whitley, R. J., Nahmias, A., Lewin, E. B., Linneman, C. C., Frenkel, L. D., Bellanti, J. A., Buchanan, R. A., Alford, C. A.: "Antiviral chemotherapy and neonatal herpes simplex virus infection: a pilot study — experience with adenin arabinoside (ARA-A)" *Pediatria 55*, 5, 678, 1975.

Chilton, N. W.: "Herpetic stomatitis. A report of six cases occurring in one family" *Am. J. Orthod. 30*, 335. 1944.

Chitwood, L. A.: "Herpesvirus infections" *Postgrad. Med. 48*, 213, 1970.

Cibis, A., Burde, R. M.: "Herpes simplex virus-induced congenital cataracts" *Acta Ophthalmol. 85*, 220, 1971.

Clark, R. M.: "Fatal systemic herpes simplex infection in a newborn infant" *Canad. Med. Assoc. J., 93*, 714, 1965.

Cleoburry, J. F., Skinner, G. R. B.: "Association between psychopathic disorder and serum antibody to herpes simplex virus (type 1)", *Brit. Med. J. 1*, 438, 1971.

Clizer, E. E., Ionnides, G.: "Herpes simplex encephalitis" *New. Eng. J. Med. 112*, 273, 1971.

143

Coetze, J. N.: "The epidemiology of herpes s'mplex in the Pretoria Bantu population" *S. Afr. J. Lab. Clin. Med. 1*, 52, 1955.

Colebatch, J. A.: "Clinical picture of severe generalised viral infection in the newborn" *Med. J. Austral. 377*, 1956.

Coleman, V. R., Thygeson, P.: "Isolation of virus from herpetic keratitis. Influence of idoxyuridine on isolation rates" *Arch. Ophthalmol. 81*, 22, 1969.

Collonello, F., Signorini, C.: "Indagini virologische sulle nevrassiti acute sporadiche in provincia di Brescia" *Gicvr. Mal. Infett. Parasit. 24*, 777, 1972.

Collory, E. V.: "The problem of intranuclear inclusions in virus diseases" *Arch. Path. 18*, 527, 1934.

Constantine, V. S., Francis, R. D., Montes, L. F.: "Association of recurrent herpes simplex with neuralgia" *JAMA 205*, 3, 131, 1968.

Coons, A. H., Snyder, J. C., Sheever, F. S.: "Localization of antigen in tissue cells" *J. Exper. Med. 91*, 31, 1950.

Cooper, M. D., Chase, H. P., Lowman, J. T., Krivit, W., Good, R. A.: "'Wiscot'-Aldrich syndrome' in immunological deficiency disease involving the afferent limb of immunity" *Am. J. Med. 44*, 499, 1968.

Copaitich, T., Turbesi, G., Traditi, F., Ugolini, A.: "Epidemia familiare d gingivo-stomatite erpetica. Aspetti clinici e immunologici" *Giorn. Mal. Infett. Parasit. 24*, 783, 1972.

Corbett, M. B., Sidell, G. M., Zimmerman, M.: "Idoxyuridine in the treatment of cutaneous herpes simplex" *JAMA 196*, 411, 1966.

Corwin, M. E., Tanne, E.: "Cryotherapy in experimental herpes simplex keratitis" *Am. J. Ophthalmol. 70*, 33, 1970.

Craig, C. P., Nahmias, A. J.: Abstr. 11-th Intersc. Conf. Antimicr. Agents and Chemoth. Atlantic City, New Jersey, Oct. 19—22, 1971.

Craig, C. P., Nahmias, A. J.: "Different patterns of neurologic involvement with HV types 1 and 2: isolation of HV type 2 from buffy coat of two adults with meningitis" *J. Infect. Dis. 127*, 365, 1973.

Crausaz, G.: "Meningoencephalite herpètique" *Rev. Med. 12*, 899, 1972.

Crosby, D. I., Henry Jores, J., Sussman, M.: "Herpetic naso-oral ulcers after renal transplantation" — *Lancet*, 2, 1191, 1969.

Cushing, H.: "The surgical aspects of major neuralgia of trigeminal nerve: report of twenty cases of operation on Gasserian ganglion, with anatomic and physiologic consequences of its removal" *JAMA 44*, 773 (1905), (cit. by Constantine *et al.* 1968).

Daniels, C., A., Borsos, T., Rapp, A., Snyderman, R., Notkins, A. L.: "Neutralization of sensitized virus by purified components of complement" *Proc. Natl. Acad. Sci. USA 65*, 528, 1970.

Daniels, C. A., LeGoff, S. G., Notkins, A. L.: "Shedding of infectious virus antibody complexes from vesicular lesions of patients with recurrent herpes labialis" *Lancet 2*, 524, 1975.

Dano, G.: "Acute cerebellar ataxia associated with herpes simplex infection" *Acta Paediatr. Scand. 57*, 151, 1968.

Darlington, R. W., Granoff, A.: "Replication: biological aspects," in Kaplan, A. S. *The herpesviruses* (Academic Press, New York, 1973).

Davidson, S. I., Evans, P. J.: "IDU and the treatment of herpes simplex keratitis" *Brit. J. Ophthalmol. 48*, 678, 1964.

144

Dayan, A. D., Lewis, P. D.: "Idoxyuridine and jaundice" *Lancet 2*, 1073, 1969.

Dayan, A. D., Goddy, W., Harrison, M. J. G., Rudge, P.: "Brain stem encephalitis caused by herpes virus hominis" *Brit. J. Med. 18*, 405, 1972.

Dayan, A. D., Stokes, M. I.: "Rapid diagnosis of encephalitis by immunofluorescent examination of cerebrospinal fluid" *Lancet 2*, 177, 1973.

Dawson, J. R.: "Cellular inclusions in the cerebral lesions of lethargic encephalitis" *Amer. J. Path. 9*, 7, 1933.

Dean, A. G., Williams, E. H., Attobua, C., Cadi, A., Omeda, J., Amuti, A. Atima, S. B.: "Clinical events suggesting herpes simplex infection before onset of Burkitt's lymphoma" *Lancet 2*, 1225, 1973.

Debré, R.: "L'herpès grave" *Strasbourg Med. 9*, 721, 1958.

Debré, R., Mozziconacci, P., Habib, R., Gautier, M., Rivron, E.: "Herpès généralisé mortel du nouveau-né" *Arch. Fr. Pediatr. 12*, 441, 1955.

De Clercq, E., Merigan, T. C.: "Current concepts of interferon and interferon induction" *Ann. Rev. Med. 21*, 17, 1970.

De Clercq, E., Edi, V. G., De Vlieger, H., Eeckels, R., Desmyter, J.: "Intratecal administration of interferon in neonatal herpes" *J. Ped. 5*, 736, 1975.

Diderholm, H., Sternram, U., Tegner, K. B., Willén, R.: "Herpes simplex hepatitis in adult" *Acta Med. Scand. 186*, 151, 1969.

Dodd, K., Johnson, M. L., Buddingh, G. J.: "Herpetic stomatitis" *J. Ped. 12*, 95, 1938.

Doden, W., Lieb, W., Wacker, A.: "Herpes corneae: Therapie mit Interferoninduktoren" *Ber. Deutch. Ophthalmol. Ges. 70*, 434, 1970.

Dodge, P. R., Cure, C. W.: "Acute encephalitis with intranuclear cellular inclusions: a neonatal case of probable herpetic etiology diagnosed by biopsy" *N. Eng. J. Med. 255*, 849, 1956.

Doeglas, H. M. G., Moolhuysen, M. G. F.: "Kaposi's varicelliform eruptione" *Arch. Dermatol. 100*, 592, 1969.

Dölle, W.: "Herpes simplex-Hepatitis beim Erwachsenen" *Internist. 13*, 465, 1972.

Döpper, T., Spaar, F. W.: "Radiologische Befund bei herpes simplex encephalitis" *Fortschr. Geb. Roentgenstr. Nuklearmed. 114*, 463, 1971.

Douglas, R. G., Anderson, S. W., Weg, J. G., Williams, T., Jenkins, D. E., Knight, V., Beall, A. C.: "Herpes simplex virus pneumonia" *JAMA 210*, 902, 1969.

Douglas, R. G., Couch, R. B.: "A prospective study of chronic herpes simplex virus infection and recurrent herpes labialis in humans" *J. Immunol. 104*, 289, 1970.

Dowdle, W., Nahmias, A. J., Harwell, R., Pauls, F.: "Association of antigenic type of herpes-virus hominis to site of viral recovery" *J. Immunol. 99*, 974, 1967.

Drachman, D. A., Adams. R. D.: "Herpes simplex and acute inclusion-body encephalitis" *Arch. Neurol. 7*, 45, 1962.

Dubois-Dalcq, M., Buyse, M., Le Febure, N., Sprecher-Goldberger, S.: "Herpesvirus hominis type 2 and intranculear tubular structures in organized nervous tissue cultures" *Acta Neuropath. 22*, 170, 1972.

Duenas, A., Adam, E., Melnick, J. L., Rawls, W. E.: "Herpesvirus type 2 in a prostitute population" *Am. J. Epidemiol. 95*, 483, 1972.

Duxbury, A. E., Lawrence, J. R.: "Primary venereal herpes simplex infection in the male" *Med. J. Austral 2*, 250, 1959.

Merinkangas, U. R., Binlou, C. O., Brutton, O. C., Trask, S. G., M.: "Skin infections in wrestlers due to herpes simplex virus" 4, 9, 1001, 1965.

Dy. .ker, Y.: "Effect of p-fluorophenylalanine on the replication of herpes simplex virus" Israeli J. Med. Sci. 5, 1083, 1969.

Echeverria, P., Miller, G., Campbell, A. G. M., Tucker, G.: "Scalp vesicles within the first week of life a clue to early diagnosis of herpes neonatorum" J. Pediatr. 83, 6, 1062, 1973.

Epstein, H. C., Crouch, W. L.: "Herpes simplex of the newborn infant" Pediatrics 13, 553, 1954.

Epstein, M. A.: "Observations on the fine structure of mature herpes simplex virus and on the composition of its nucleoid" J. Exp. Med. 115, 1, 1962.

Epstein, M. A.: "Human putative oncogenic herpesviruses" in ed. Clemmesen, J. and Yohn, D. S., "Comparative leukemia research" Bibliot. Haemat., N. 43, pp. 318—321, (Karger, Basel, 1976).

Epstein, M. A., Barr, Y. M., Achong, B. C.: "Studies with Burkitt's lymphoma" Wistar Inst. Symp. Monogr. 4, 69, 1965.

Ericsson, H., Ivemark, B. I., Johnsson, T., Zetterström, R.: "Generalised herpes simplex infection associated with staphylococcal septicemia in a newborn infant" Acta Paediatr. 47, 666, 1958.

Esser, M.: "Ueber eine kleine Epidemie von Pustulosis varioliformis acuta" Ann. Paediatr. 157, 156, 1941.

Evans, A. D., Gray, O. P., Miller, M. N.: "Herpes simplex encephalitis treated with intravenous idoxyuridine" Brit. Med. J. 2, 407, 1967.

Evans, A. D., Holzel, A.: "Immune deficiency state in a girl with eczema and low serum IgM" Arch. Dis. Child. 45, 527, 1970.

Falke, B., Heicke, B., Bässler, R.: "The effect of arabinofuranosulcytosine upon the synthesis of herpesvirus hominis" Arch. ges. Virusforsch 39, 48, 1972.

Falke, D., Rada, B.: "6-Azauridine as an inhibitor of the synthesis of herpesvirus hominis" Acta Virol. 14, 115—23, 1970.

Falke, D., Kahl, L.: "The inhibitory effect of compound 48/90 on the formation of giant cells induced by herpes virus hominis" J. Gen. Virol. 10, 273, 1971.

Felber, T. D.: "Photoinactivation may find use against herpesvirus" JAMA 217, 270, 1971.

Felber, T. D., Smith, E. B., Knox, J. M., Wallis, C., Melnick, L.: "Photodynamic inactivation of herpes simplex" JAMA 223, 289, 1973.

Felder, J., Mühlethaler, J. P., Krach, U.: "Herpes simplex generalisatus eigener fall and kasuistischer Uberblick" Helv. Paediatr. Acta 5, 451, 1960.

Felsburg, P. J., Heberling, R. L., Kalter, S. S.: "Experimental genital infection of cebus monkeys with oral and genital isolates of herpesvirus hominis type 1 and 2" Arch. ges. Virusforsch. 39, 223, 1972.

Fiala, M., Chow, A. W., Miyasaki, K., Guze, L. B.: "Susceptibility of herpes virus to cytosine arabinoside (ara-C)" Bacteriol. Proc. 225, 1972.

Fiala, M., Chow, A., Guze, L. B.: "Susceptibility of herpesviruses to cytosine arabinoside: standardization of susceptibility test procedure and relative resistance of herpes simplex type 2 strains" *Antimicrob. Agents. Chemother 354,* 1971, 1972.

Fiala, M., Chow, A., Miyasaki, K., Guze, L. B.: "Susceptibility of herpesviruses to three nucleotide analogues and their combinations and enhancement of the antiviral effect at acid pH" *J. Infect. Dis. 129,* 1, 82, 1974.

Field, A. K., Tytell, A., Lampson, G. P., Hilleman, M. R.: "Inducers of interferon and host response. II Multistranded synthetic polynucleotide complexes" *Proc. Natl. Acad. Sci. 58,* 1004, 1967.

Findlay, G. M., MacCallum, F. O.: "Recurrent traumatic herpes" *Lancet 1,* 259, 1940.

Fingerland, A., Toušek, M.: "Encephalitis herpetica" *Čas. Lek. Česk. 89,* 18, 1950.

Fingerland, A., Vortel, V., Endrys, J.: "Esophagitis herpetica" *Čas. Lek. Česk. 91,* 473, 1952.

Finelli, P. F., Mc Donald, S. D.: "Herpe s simplex virus in sensory ganglions" *New Engl. J. Med., 292,* 51, 1975.

Fisher, B. K., Kibrick, S.: "Primary herpes in adult with Darier's disease" *Arch. Dermatol. 87,* 229, 1963.

Flewett, T. H., Parker, R. G. F., Philip, W. M.: "Acute hepatitis due to herpes simplex virus in an adult" *J. Clin. Pathol. 22,* 60, 1969.

Florman, A. L., Mindlin, R. L.: "Generalized herpes simplex in an eleven-day-old premature infant" *Am. J. Dis. Child. 83,* 481, 1952.

Florman, A. L., Gershon, A. A., Blackett, P. R., Nahmias, A. J.: "Intrauterine infection with herpes simplex virus" *JAMA 225,* 129, 1973.

Foerster, D. W., Scott, L. V.: "Isolation of herpes simplex from a patient with erythema multiforme exudativum (Stevens-Johnson syndrome)" *New Eng. J. Med. 259,* 473, 1958.

Foley, F. D., Greenawald, K. A., Nash, G., Pruitt, B. A.: "Herpes virus infection in burned patients" *New Eng. J. Med. 12,* 652, 1970.

Forman, L., Whitwell, G. P. B.: "Association of herpes catarrhalis with erythema multiforme (hebra)" *Brit. J. Dermatol. Syph. 46,* 309, 1934.

France, N. E., Wilmers, M. J.: "Herpes simplex hepatitis and encephalitis in newborn twins" *Lancet 1,* 1181, 1953.

Francis, D. P., Herrman, K. L., MacMahon, J. R., Chavingy, K. H., Sanderlin, K. C.: "Nosocomial and maternally acquired herpesvirus hominis infection" *Am. J. Dis. Child. 129,* 889, 1975.

Francis, T. I., Osuntokun, B. O., Kemp, G. E.: "Fulminant hepatitis due to herpes hominis in an adult human" *Am. J. Gastroenterol. 57,* 329, 1972.

Frangini, V., Matucci, C. L.: "Malattia erpetica neonatale" *Ric. Clin. Pediatr., 84,* 118, 1971.

Frenkel, N., Roizman, B., Casai, E., Nahmias, A. J: "A herpes simplex 2 DNA fragment: its transcription in human cervical cancer tissue" *Proc. Natl. Acad. Sci., 69,* 3784, 1972.

Frenz, J. M., Gohd, R. S., Woody, N. C.: "Untreated neonatal herpes simplex, 2 meningitis without apparent neurologic damage" *J. Pediatr. 85,* 77 1974.

Freund, H.: "Uber den Nachweis des Herpes Erregers bei zosteriformen Eruptionen (Darier) und sein differential diagnostische Bedeutung" *Arch. Dermatol. Syph. 154,* 278, 1928.

Freund, H.: "Zur Aetiologie der Pustulosis vacciniformis acuta (Kaposi-Juliusberg)" *Dermatol. Wschr. 98,* 2, 58, 1934.

Frezzotti, T., Guerra, R.: "Malattie oculari da herpes virus (virus dell'herpes simplex, dell'herpes zoster-varicella)" *Gior. Malatt. Infett. Parass. 7,* 689, 1971.

Friedrich, E. G.: "Relief for herpes vulvitis" *Obstet. Gynecol. 41,* 74, 1973.

Fruitstone, M. J., Waddell, G. H., Sigel, M.: "An interferon produced in response to infection by herpes simplex virus" *Proc. Soc. Exp. Biol. Med. 117,* 804, 1964.

Gagnon, R.: "Transplancental inoculation of fatal herpes simplex in the newborn. Report of two cases" *Obstet. Gynecol. 31,* 682, 1968.

Galagher, W. F.: "Burn-wound infection with viruses" *New Eng. J. Med. 282,* 1272, 1970.

Gardner, P. S., McQuillin, J., Black, M. M., Richardson, J.: "Rapid diagnosis of herpes virus hominis infections in superficial lesions by immunofluorescent antibody techniques" *Brit. Med. J. 4,* 89, 1968.

Gerber, P., Rosenblum, E. N.: "The incidence of complement-fixing antibodies to herpes simplex and herpes-like viruses in man and rhesus monkeys" *Proc. Soc. Exp. Biol. Med. 128,* 541, 1968.

Gerola, M.: "Malattia connatale da herpes virus hominis" nel "Malattie neonatali ad incorgenza nella vita fetale" Atti dell XXXV Congresso della Società Italiana — Verona, 1972. Di Pediatria Ed. Minerva Ped. Torino.

Gershon, A. A., Fish, I., Brunell, P. A.: "Herpes simplex infection of the newborn" *Am. J. Dis. Child. 124,* 739, 1972.

Gilbert, D. N., Johnson, M. T., Luby, J. P., Stanford, J. P.: "Herpes virus hominis type 1 encephalitis treated with cytarabine an unresolved problem in encephalitis" *Medicine 52,* 331, 1972.

Gillot, F., Schaefer, J. C., Dalaut, J. J.: "La maladie herpètique du nourrisson et ses limites (a propos d'un cas)" *Presse Mèd. 66,* 307 1958.

Ginder, D. R., Whorten, C. M.: "Herpes simplex encephalitis" *J. Pediatr. 39,* 298, 1951.

Glezen, W. P., Fernald, G. W., Lohr, J. A.: "Acute respiratory disease of university students with special reference to the etiologic role of herpesvirus hominis" *Am. J. Epidemiol. 101,* 2, 111, 1975.

Gold, J. A., Stewart, R. C., McKee, J.: "The epidemiology and chemotherapy of herpes simplex keratitis and herpes simplex skin infections" *Ann. NY. Acad Sci. 130,* 209, 1965.

Golden, B., Bell, W. E., McKee, A. P.: "Disseminated herpes simplex with encephalitis in a neonate. Treatment with idoxyuridine" *JAMA 209,* 1219, 1969.

Goldman, J. M., Goodman, M. L., Miler, D.: "Antibody to Epstein-Barr virus in American patients with carcinoma of the nasospharynx" *JAMA 216,* 1618, 1971.

Goldman, L.: "Reactions of autoinoculation for recurrent herpes simplex" *Arch. Dermatol.* 84, 1025, 1961.

Goldman, R. L.: "Herpetic inclusions in the endometrium" *Obstet. Gynecol. 36,* 603, 1970.

Gompertz, C.: "Prospects for radiation treatment of herpetic and other affections of the anterior segment of the eye" *Ophthalmologica 155,* 130, 1968.

Good, R. A., Campbell, B.: "The precipitation of latent herpes simplex encephalitis by anaphylactic shock" *Proc. Soc. Exp. Biol. Med. 59,* 305, 1945.

Goodheart, C. R.: "Herpesvirus and cancer" *JAMA 211,* 1, 91, 1970.

148

Goodpasture, E. W., Teague, O.: "Transmission of the virus herpes febrilis along nerves in experimentally infected rabbits" *J. Med. Res. 44*, 139, 1923.

Gostling, J. V. T.: "Viral diseases of the nervous system: herpetic encephalitis" *Proc. Roy. Soc. Med. 60*, 21, 1967.

Goyette, R. E., Donowho, E. M., Hieger, L. R., Planherr, G. D.: "Fulminant herpesvirus hepatitis during pregnancy" *Obstet. Gynecol. 43*, 191, 1974.

Graciansky, P., Timsit, E., Martinet, C.: "Pustulose de Kaposi-Juliusberg par primo-infection herpètique chez un adulte attient d'eczema constitutionnel" *Arch. Belg. Dermatol. Syph. 26*, 255, 1970.

Grant, H. E., McMenemey, W. H.: "Encephalitides" in L. Van Bogaert *et al.*, eds. *Proceedings of a symposium on the neuropathology, electroencephalography and biochemistry of encephalitides, Antwerp, 1959* (Elsevier) Amsterdam, 1961, pp. 227—229.

Graupner, K., Muller, F.: "Zur Behandlung der Keratitis dendritica mit parafluorphenylalanin" *Arch. Ophthalmol. 174*, 231, 1968.

Green, L. H., Levin, M. P.: "An unusal primary infection with herpes simplex virus: a case report" *J. Periodont 42*, 170, 1971.

Griffith, J. F., Fitzwilliam, J. F., Casagrande, S., Butler, R. S.: "Experimental herpes simplex virus encephalitis: comparative effects of treatment with cytosine arabinoside and adenine arabinoside" *J. Infect. Dis. 132*, 5, 506, 1975.

Grüter, W.: "Experimentalle und klinische Untersuchungen uber den sogenannten Herpes corneae" *Ber. Deutsch. Ophthalmol. Ges. 42*, 162, 1920.

Gudnadottir, M., Helgadottir, H., Bjarnason, O., Jonsdottir, K.: "Virus isolated from the brain of a patient with multiple sclerosis" *Exp. Neurol. 9*, 85, 1964.

Guerra, R., Frezzotti, R., Bonanni, R., Dianzanti, F., Rita, C.: "A preliminary study on the treatment of human herpes simplex keratitis with an interferon inducer" *Ann. N. Y. Acad. Sci. 173*, 823, 1970.

Guha, D. K., Rashmi, A., Khanduja, P. C.: "In utero infection of the fetus by herpes simplex virus" *Indian J. Pediatr. 35*, 484, 1968.

Gundersen, I. T.: "Herpes corneae with special reference to its treatment with a strong solution of iodine" *Arch. Ophthalmol. 15*, 225, 1936.

Hader, W., Bawatpour, M., Dempster, G., Rozdilsky, B.: "Herpes simplex encephalitis: two fatal cases" *Canad. Med. Assoc. J. 96*, 1565, 1967.

Hagler, W. S., Walters, P. V., Nahmias, A. J.: "Ocular involvement in neonatal herpes simplex virus infection" *Arch. Ophthalmol. 82*, 168, 1969.

Hale, B. D., Rentdorff, R. C., Walker, L. C.: "Epidemic herpetic stomatitis in an orphanage nursery" *JAMA 183*, 1068, 1963.

Hall-Smith, S. P., Corrigan, M. J., Gilkes, M. J.: "Treatment of herpes simplex with 5-iodo-deoxyuridine" *Br. Med. J. 1515*, 1962.

Hambrick, G. W., Cox, R. P.: "Primary herpes simplex infections of fingers of medical personnel" *Arch. Dermatol. 85*, 583, 1962.

Hamilton, L. D., Babcock, V. I., Southam, C. M.: "Inhibition of herpes simplex virus by synthetic double-stranded RNA (polyriboadenylic and polyribouridylic acids and polyriboinosinic and polyribocydylic acids)" *Microbiology 64*, 778, 1969.

Hamory, B. C., Osterman, C. A., Wenzel, R. P.: "Herpetic whitlow" *New Eng. J. Med. 292*, 268, 1975.

Hampar, B., Notkins, A. L., Mage, M., Keehn, M. A.: "Heterogeneity in the properties of 75 and 19 S rabbit neutralizing antibodies to herpes simplex virus" *J. Immunol. 100*, 586, 1968a.

Hampar, B., Mage, M., Keehn, M. A.: "Heterogeneity in the ability of rabbit 7 S and 19 S neutralizing antibodies to differentiate between intratypic antigenic variants of herpes simplex virus" *J. Immunol. 101*, 256, 1968b.

Hampar, B., Martos, L. M., Chakrabarty, M., Burroughs, M. A. K.: "Late 19 S rabbit antibody neutralization test for differentiating herpes simplex virus types 1 and 2" *J. Immunol. 104*, 593, 1970.

Hampar, B., Miyamoto, K., Martos, L. M.: "Serologic classification of herpes simplex viruses" *J. Immunol. 106*, 580, 1971a.

Hampar, B., Hsu, K. C., Martos, L. M., Walker, J. L.: "Serologic evidence that a herpes-type virus is the etiologic agent of heterophyle-positive infectious mononucleosis" *Proc. Natl. Acad. Sci. 68*, 7, 1407, 1971b.

Hanna, L., Jawetz, E., Coleman, V. R.: "Studies on herpes simplex VIII. The significance of isolating herpes simplex virus from the eye" *Am. J. Ophthalmol. 43*, 126, 1957.

Hansen, J. D. L.: "Herpes simplex stomatitis in children: its clinical picture and complication as seen in Cape Town" *S. Afr. Med. J. 35*, 131, 1961.

Hanshaw, J. B.: "Idoxuridine in herpes virus encephalitis" *N. Eng. J. Med. 282*, 47, 1969.

Harland, W. A., Adams, J. H., McSeveney, D.: "Herpes simplex particles in acute necrotizing encephalitis" *Lancet 1*, 581, 1967.

Hass, G. M.: "Hepato-adrenal necrosis with intranuclear inclusion bodies: report of a case" *Am. J. Pathol. 11*, 127, 1935.

Hathaway, W. E., Mull, M. M., Pechet, G. S.: "Disseminated intravascular coagulation in the newborn" *Pediatrics 43*, 233, 1969.

Haynes, R. E.: "Treatment of herpes virus encephalitis with iododeoxyuridine" *J. Pediatr. 83*, 102, 1973.

Haynes, R. E., Azimi, P. H., Gramblett, H. G.: "Fatal herpesvirus hominis (herpes simplex virus) infections in children" *JAMA 206*, 2, 312, 1968.

Haymaker, W.: "Herpes simplex encephalitis in man: with a report of three cases" *J. Neuropathol. Exp. Neurol. 8*, 132, 1949.

Haymaker, W., Smith, M. G., van Bogeart, L.: "Pathology of viral disease in man characterized by nuclear inclusions with emphasis on herpes simplex and subacute inclusion ecephalitis in W. S. Fields and R. J. Blattner, eds., *Viral. encepalitis* (Springfield, Ill., 1959), p. 95.

Henle, G., Henle, W.: "Immunofluorescence interference and complement fixation techniques in the detection of the herpes type virus in Burkitt tumor cell lines" *Cancer Res. 27*, 2442, 1967.

Henle, G., Henle, W., Diehl, V.: "Relation of Burkitt's tumor associated herpes type virus to infectious mononucleosis" *Proc. Natl. Acad. Sci. 59*, 94, 1968.

Henle, W., Henle, G., Ho, H. C., Burtin, B., Cachin, Y., Cliford, P., De Schryver, A., De The, G., Diehl, V.: "Antibodies to Epstein-Barr virus in nasopharyngeal carcinoma, other head and neck neoplasms and control groups" *J. Natl. Cancer. Inst. 44*, 225, 1970.

Hènocq, E.: "Actualité du vaccin anti-herpètique" *Thèrapeutique 48*, 485, 1972.

Herout, V., Vortel, V., Vondračkova, A.: "Herpes simplex involvement of the lower respiratory tract" *Am. J. Clin. Pathol. 46*, 4, 411, 1966.

Heyne, K.: "Granulozyten-Nekrobiose bei generalisierter Herpes-simplex-Virus Infection des Neugeborenen" *Helv. Paediatr. Acta. 29*, 127, 1974.

Hirsch, M. S., Gary, G. W., Murphy, F. A.: "In vitro and in vivo properties of antimacrophage sera" *J. Immunol. 102*, 656, 1969.

Hirsch, M. S., Zisman, B., Allison, A. C.: "Macrophages and age-dependent resistance to herpes simplex virus in mice" *J. Immunol. 104*, 1160, 1970.

Hirschaut, Y., Glede, P., Octavio, L., Vieira, B. D., Aibender, E., Dvorak, B., Siltzbach, L. E.: "Sarcoidosis, another disease associated with serologic evidence for herpes-like virus infection" *New Eng. J. Med. 283*, 502, 1970.

Hitselberg, J. F., Burns, R. F.: "Darier's disease report of a case complicated by Kaposi's varicelliform eruption" *Arch. Dermatol. 83*, 425, 1968.

Holzel, A., Feldman, G. V., Tobin, J. O. H., Harper, J.: "Herpes simplex: a study of complement fixing antibodies at different ages" *Acta Paediatr. 42*, 206, 1953.

Hovig, D. E., Hodgman, J. E., Mathies, A. W.: "Herpes virus hominis (simplex) infection" *Am. J. Dis. Child. 115*, 438, 1968.

Howard, R. C.: "Herpes simplex keratoconjunctivitis" *Am. J. Ophthalmol. 62*, 907, 1966.

Hudson, A. W., McFarland, C.: "Disseminated herpes simplex in the newborn. A consequence of infection in the mother" *JAMA 208*, 859, 1969.

Hughes, J. T.,: "Pathology of herpes simplex encephalitis" in Whitty, C. W., et al., eds., *Virus diseases and the nervous system* (Blackwell, Oxford, 1969).

Hughes, W. F.: "Treatment of herpes simplex keratitis" *Am. J. Ophthalmol., 67*, 313, 1969.

Hunt, B. P., Comer, E. B. O.: "Herpetic meningoencephalitis accompanying cutaneous herpes simplex" *Am. J. Med. 19*, 814, 1955.

Hutfield, D. C.: "Fatal effects of herpes genitalis on the newborn infant" *J. Gynecol. Obstet. Brit. Cwlth. 73*, 1020, 1966a.

Hutfield, D. C.: "History of herpes genitalis" *Brit. J. Vener. Dis. 42*, 263ᵧ 1966b.

Hutfield, D. C.: "Herpes genitalis" *Brit. J. Vener. Dis. 44*, 241, 1968.

Hutton, R. D., Stegman, S. J.: "Herpes simplex of penis and anus" *Arch. Dermatol. 108*, 580, 1973.

Ikić, D., Smerdel, A., Šoš, E., Jelušić, D.: "Imunological protection and therapy of human genital herpes" *Rad. Imunol. zavoda, Zagreb 13*, 113, 1971.

Illis, L. S., Taylor, F. M.: "The electroencephalogram in herpes simplex encephalitis" *Lancet 1*, 718, 1972.

Indgin, S. N., Connor, J. D.: "Pemphigus and herpes simplex" *Arch. Dermatol. 102*, 333, 1970.

Isaacs, A.: "Nature and functions of interferon" in Pollard, ed., *Prospectives in virology* (Burge, Minneapolis, 1961.).

Ito, Y., Takahashi, T., Tu, S., Kawamura, Jr., A.: "High anti EB virus titer in sera of patients with nasopharyngeal carcinoma: a small scaled seroepidemiological study" *Gann. 60*, 334, 1969.

Ive, F. A.: "A trial of 5-iodo-2-deoxyuridine in herpes simplex" *Brit. J. Dermatol. 76*, 463-4, 1964.

Iwanami, K., Irino, T., Hamamoto, Y.: "An autopsy case of visceral herpes simplex in a neonatal infant" *Bull. Osaka Med. Sch. 14*, 25, 1968.

Izumi, A., Goldschmidt, H.: "Herpes simplex infection complicating Darier's disease" *Arch. Dermatol. 102*, 650, 1970.

151

Jack, I., Perry, J. W.: "Herpes simplex infection in the newborn" *Med. J. Austral.* *46*, 640, 1959.

JAMA *217*, 270, 1971. Medical news: "Photoinactivation may find use against herpesvirus."

JAMA *230*, 2, 189, 1974. Medical news: "A review of preliminary results of adenine arabinoside studies."

Janbon, M., Chaptal, J., Labraque-Bordanave, M.: "Le probleme de la meningite herpetique: contribution a son etude clinique et experimentale" *Presse Med.* *50*, 145, 1942.

Jank, M., Söltz-Szötz, J.: "Zur Immunologie des Eczema herpetiforme Kaposi" *Hautarzt*, *17*, 163, 1966.

Jawetz, E.: "Chemotherapy of herpesviruses: clinical aspects" p. 665—685 in Kaplan, A. S. ed., *The Herpesviruses* (Academic Press, New York, 1973).

Jawetz, E., Coleman, V. R., Dawson, C. R., Thygeson, P.: "The dynamics of IUDR action in herpetic keratitis and the emergence of IUDR resistance in vivo" *Ann. N. Y. Acad. Sci.* *173*, 282, 1970.

Jeansson, S., Molin, L.: "Genital herpes infection and nonspecific urethritis" *Brit. Med. J.* 2, 247, 1971.

Jelić, O., Kovačević, Lj., Čubelić, P.: "Prikaz bolesnika s akutnim meningoencefalitisom u toku visceralne herpes simpleks infekcije" (Acute meningoencephalitis in the course of disseminated herpesvirus infection) *Jug. Pediatr.* *16*, 187, 1973.

Jensen, J., Snyderman, R., Mergenhagen, S., in H. Movat, ed., *Cellular and humoral mechanisms in anaphylaxis and allergy* (Karger, Basel, 1969), p. 265.

Johnson, A. G., Gone, R. E., Friedman, H. M., Han, I. H., Johnson, H. G., Smichmidtke, J. R., Stout, R. D., in R. Beers and W. Brown, eds., *Biological Effects of Polynucleotides* (Springer, New York, 1971), p. 52.

Johnson, R. T.: "The pathogenesis of herpes simplex encephalitis, I, Virus pathways to the nervous system of suckling mice demonstrated by fluorescent antibody staining" *J. Exp. Med.,* *119*, 343, 1964a.

Johnson, R. T.: "The pathogenesis of herpes simplex encephalitis" *J. Exp. Med.,* *120*, 359, 1964b.

Johnson, R. T., Mims, C. A.: "Pathogenesis of viral infections of the nervous system" *New Eng. J. Med.* *278*, 84, 1968.

Johnson, R. T., Olson, L. C.: "Herpes simplex virus infections of the nervous system" *Arch. Psychiat.* *18*, 260, 1969.

Josey, W. E.: "Summary of informal discussion of part I of genital herpesvirus" *Cancer Res.* *33*, 1464, 1973.

Josey, W. E., Nahmias, A. J., Naib, Z. M., Utley, P. M., McKenzie, W. J., Coleman, M. T.: "Genital herpes infection in the female" *Am. J. Obstet. Gynecol.* *96*, 493, 1966.

Josey, W. E., Nahmias, A. J., Naib, Z. M.: "Genital infection with type 2 herpesvirus hominis: present knowledge and possible relation to cervical cancer" *Am. J. Obstet. Gynecol.* *101*, 718, 1968.

Juel-Jensen, B. E.: "Severe generalized primary herpes treated with cytarabine" *Brit. Med. J.* 2, 154, 1970.

Juel-Jensen, B. E., MacCallum, F. O.: "Treatment of herpes simplex lesions of the face with idoxyridine: results of a double blind controlled trial" *Brit. Med. J.* 2, 987—8, 1964.

Juretić, M.: "Incubation period of primary herpetic infection" *Helv. Peadiatr. Acta 15*, 102, 1960.

152

Juretić, M.: "Natural history of herpetic infection" *Helv. Paediatr. Acta 21*, 356, 1966.

Juretić, M.: "Primarna herpetična infekcija" (Primary herpetic infection) *Izd. Zavoda za zaštitu zdravlja Rijeka*, 1970.

Juretić, M., Brož, M.: "Epidemije herpetičke infekcije" (Epidemics of herpetic infections) *Jug. Pediatr. 1*, 1960.

Juretić, M., Petković, B.: "Prilog epidemilogiji primarne herpetične infekcije" (A contribution to the epidemiology of primary herpetic infection) *Liječ. Vjesn. 5*, 383, 1960.

Juretić, M., Rajh, M.: "Primarna herpetična infekcija kod djeteta sa dermatitis ammoniacalis" (Primary herpetic infection in a child with dermatitis ammoniacalis) *ZMD 20*, 229, 1976.

Juretić, M., Ribarić, V.: "Iodoxiuridine u profilaksi eksperimentalne herpetične infekcije" (Iodoxyuridine in the prophylaxis of experimential herpetic infection) *Jug. Ped. 13*, 67, 1970.

Juretić, M., Katunarić, B., Puretić, S., Puretić, B.: "Erythema exudativum multiforme maius" *Liječ. Vjesn.* 86, 911, 1964.

Kalter, S. S., Felsburg, P. J., Heberling, R. L.: Experimental herpesvirus hominis type 2 infection of monkeys" *Proc. Soc. Exp. Biol. 139*, 964, 1972.

Kanaar, P.: "Primary herpes simplex infections of fingers in nurses" *Dermatologica 134*, 346, 1967.

Kaplan, A. S., ed.: The herpesviruses (Academic Press, New York, 1973).

Kaposi, M. J.: Pathologie und Therapie der Hautkrankeiten (Urban & Schwarzenberg, Berlin, 1887).

Kaufman, H. E.: "Chemotherapy of virus disease" *Chemotherapia* 7, 1, 1963.

Kaufman, H. E.: "Local immunity" *Arch. Ophthalmol. 83*, 131, 1970.

Kaufman, H. E., Maloney, E. D.: "IDU and cytosine arabinoside in experimental herpetic keratitis" *Arch. Ophthalmol. 69*, 626, 1963.

Kaufman, H. E., Nesburn, A. B., Maloney, E. D.: "IDU therapy of herpes simplex keratitis" *Arch. Ophthalmol., 67*, 583, 1962.

Kaufman, H. E., Martola, E., Dohlman, C. H.: "Herpes simplex treatment with IDU and corticosteroids" *Arch. Ophthalmol., 69*, 468, 1963.

Kaufman, H. E., Brown, D. C., Ellison, E. M.: "Recurrent herpes in rabbit and man" *Science 156*, 1628, 1967.

Kaufman, H. E., Brown, D. C., Ellison, E. M.: "Herpes virus in the lacrimal gland, conjunctiva and cornea of man. A chronic infection" *Am. J. Ophthalmol. 65*, 32, 1968.

Kaufman, H. E., Ellison, E. D., Waltman, S. R.: "Double stranded RNA and interferon inducer in herpes simplex keratitis" *Am. J. Ophthalmol., 68*, 468, 1969.

Kaufman, H. E., Kanai, A., Ellison, E. D.: "Herpes iritis: demonstration of virus in the anterior chamber by flourescent antibody techniques and electron microscopy" *Am. J. Ophthalmol.* 71, 465, 1971.

Kaufman, R. H., Melnick, J. L.: "Genital herpes in two social groups" *Am. J. Obstet. Gynecol., 110*, 683, 1971.

Kaufman, R. H., Rawls, W. H.: "Extragenital type 2 herpesvirus infection" *Am. J. Obstet. Gynecol. 112*, 866, 1972.

Kaufman, R. H., Gardner, H. L., Rawls, W. E., Dixon, R. E., Young, R. L.: "Clinical features of herpes genitalis" *Cancer Res. 33*, 1446, 1973a.

Kaufman, R. H., Gardner, H. L., Brown, D., Walls, C., Rawls, W., Melnick, J. L.: "Herpes genitalis treated by photodynamic inactivation of virus" *Am. J. Obstet. Gynecol. 117*, 1144, 1973b.

Kawai, K., Arahama, M.: "Generalized herpes simplex infection in neonatal infants. A report of two autopsy cases" *Acta Pathol. Japan. 8*, 251, 1978. (prema Iwanami).

Kawana T., Kawaguchi T., Sakamoto, S.: "Clinical and virological studies on genital herpes" *Lancet 30*, 964, 1976.

Keller, J. M., Spear, P. G., Roizman, B.: "Proteins specified by herpes simplex virus. III, Viruses differing in their effects on the social behavior of infected cells specify different membrane glycoproteins" *Proc. Natl. Acad. Sci. USA 65*, 865, 1970.

Kerenyi, N., Faulkner, R., Petite, E.: "Herpes simplex encephalitis: a fatal case" *Canad. Med. Assoc. J. 81*, 1011, 1959.

Kessler, I. I., Kulčar, Ž., Rawls, S., Smerdel, S., Strand, M., Lilienfeld, M.: "Cervical cancer in Yugoslavia. I, Antibodies to genital herpes virus in Cases and controls" *J. Natl. Canc. Inst. 52*, 362, 1974.

Kibrick, S.: "Herpes simplex," pp. 75—94 in Charls, D., and Finland, M., eds., *Obstetric and perinatal infections* (Lee & Febiger, Philadelphia, 1973).

Kibrick, S., Gooding, G. W.: "Pathogenesis of infection with herpes simplex virus with special reference to nervous tissue. Slow latent and temperate virus infections" *Monography 2*, 143, 1965.

Kilbourne, E. D., Horsfall, F. L.: "Primary herpes simplex infection of the adult with a note on the relation of herpes simplex virus to recurrent aphthous stomatitis" *Arch. Intern. Med. 88*, 495, 1951.

Kilbourne, E. D., Horsfall, F. L.: "Studies of herpes simplex. Infection in a newborn infant" *J. Lab. Clin. Med. 48*, 5742, 1951.

Kimura, S. J.: "Herpes simplex keratitis," in *Infectious Diseases of the Conjunctiva and Cornea*, Symposium of the New Orleans Academy of Ophthalmology (Mosby, St. Louis, 1963).

Kipps, A., Becker, W., Wainweight, J., McKenzie, D.: "Fatal disseminated primary herpesvirus infection in children: epidemiology based on 93 non-neonatal cases" *S. Afr. Med. J. 41*, 647, 1967.

Klastersky, J., Cappel, R., Snoeck, J. M., Flament, J., Thiry, L.: "Ascending myelitis in association with herpes simplex virus" *New Eng. J. Med. 28*, 182, 1972.

Kleger, B., Prier, J. E., Rosato, D. J., McGinnis, A. E.: "Herpes simplex infection of the female genital tract. Incidence of infection" *Am. J. Obstet. Gynecol. 102*, 745, 1968.

Klinger, M.: "Herpetička oboljenja rožnice u djece" (Herpetic disease of the cornea in children) *Archiv ZMD 5/6, 319*, 1969.

Kluge, T., Skyberg, D., Bjoro, K.: "Fatal herpes simplex infection in the newborn" *Acta. Obstet. Gynecol. Scand. 46*, 369, 1967.

Korones, S. B., Todaro, J., Roane, J. A., Sever, J. L.: "Maternal virus infection after the first trimester of pregnancy and status of offspring to 4 years of age in a predominantly Negro population" *J. Ped. 77*, 245, 1970.

Krashen, A. S.: "Cryotherapy of herpes of the mouth" *J. Am. Dent. Assoc. 81*, 1163, 1970.

Kretschmer, R., August, C. S., Rosen, F. S., Janeway, C. A.: "Recurrent infections, episodic lymphopenia and impaired cellular immunity" *New Eng. J. Med. 281*, 285, 1969.

Krueger, R. R., Mayer, G. D.: "An orally active antiviral agent: tilorone hydrochloride," *Science 169*, 1213, 1970.

154

Krugman, S.: "Primary herpetic vulvovaginitis" *Pediatrics* 9, 585, 1952.

Krwawicz, T.: "Cryogenic treatment of herpes simplex keratitis" *Brit. J. Ophthalmol.* 49, 37, 1965.

Kloene, W., Bang, F. B., Chakraborty, S. M., Cooper, M. R., Kuleman, H., Ota, M., Shah, K. V.: "A two-years respiratory survey in four villages in West Bengal, India" *Am. J. Epid.* 92, 5, 307, 1970.

Knotts, F. B., Cook, M. L., Stevens, J. G.: "Pathogenesis of herpetic encephalitis in mice after ophthalmic inoculation" *J. Inf. Dis.* 1, 16, 1974.

Krwawicz, T.: "The use of low temperature in the treatment of iridocyclitis and of herpetic infections of the cornea" *Trans. Ophthalmol. Soc. U. K.* 88, 137, 1968.

Kuchle, H. J., Kunze, B.: "Erfahrugen mit JUDR (IDU) bei Virusaffectionen der Hornhaut" *Klin. Mbl. Augenheil.* 144, 490, 1964.

Künzer, W., Majer, M., Denz, C.: "Eine ungewönlich leichte Herpes simplex Erkrankung bei einem Neugeborenen" *Deutsch. Med. Wschr.* 91, 1183, 1966.

Kurtzke, J. R.: "Inclusion body encephalitis: nonfatal case" *Neurology* 6, 371, 1956.

Kusano, N.: "Herpetic hepatitis with special reference to its transition to giant cell's hepatitis" *Acta Pathol. Japan* 10, 549, 1960.

Laboureau, J. P., Le Touze, P., Caldera, R.: "Les lesions oesophagenes dans l'herpès neonatal" *Sem. Hop. Paris* 49, 335, 1973.

Laibson, P. R.: "Cornea and sclera" *Arch. Ophthalmol.* 83, 637, 1970.

Lampson, G. P., Tyttel, A. A., Nemes, M. M., Hilleman, M. R.: "Characterization of chick embryo interferon produced by a DNA virus" *Proc. Soc. Exp. Biol. Med.* 118, 441, 1965.

Lamy, M., Jammet, M. L., Granjon, A., Vescot, J., Daniel, P., Nezelof, C., Cottin, S.: "L'herpès du nouveau-né" *Arch. Fr. Pediatr.* 17, 425, 1960.

Lancet 1, 1324, 1975: Editorial: "Can herpes simplex encephalitis be treated?"

Langvad, A., Voigt, J.: "Herpes generalisata infantum: a review and a report of a new case" *Dan. Med. Bull.* 10, 153, 1963.

Lapinleimu, K., Cantell, K., Koskimies, O., Sayen, L.: "Association between maternal herpesvirus infections and congenital malformations" *Lancet 1*, 1127, 1974.

LaRossa, D., Hamilton, R.: "Herpes simplex infection of the digits" *Arch. Surg.* 102, 602, 1971.

Lausch, R. N., Swyers, J. S., Kaufman, H. E.: "Delayed hypersensitivity to herpes simplex virus in the guinea pig" *J. Immunol.* 96, 981, 1966.

Lausecker, H.: "Zur klinik von Kaposi's varizelliformer eruption (Ekzema herpetiforme)" *Derm. Wschr.* 703, 1, 1953.

Lausecker, H.: "Des eccema herpetiforme Kaposi" *Münch. Med. Wschr.* 47 1547, 1955.

Lazar, M. D.: "Vaccination for recurrent herpes simplex infection: initiation of a new disease site following the use of unmodified material containing the live virus" *Arch. Dermatol.* 75, 70, 1956.

Lazar, P.: "Primary herpetic vulvovaginitis" *Arch. Dermatol.* 72, 272, 1955.

Leider, W., Magoffin, R. L., Mennette, E. H., Leonards, L.: "Herpes simplex virus encephalitis: its possible association with reactivated latent infection" *New Eng. J. Med.* 273, 341, 1965.

Lennette, E. H., Magoffin, R. L., Knouf, E. G.: "Viral central nervous disease; an etiological study conducted at the Los Angeles County General Hospital" *JAMA 179*, 687, 1962.

Le Tan, Vinh, Allison, F., Lelong, M.: "La maladie herpetique du nouveau--né (avec un cas personnel)" *Arch. Fr. Pediatr. 12,* 233, 1955.

Levaditi, C.: *Les ectodermoses neurotropes* (Masson, Paris, 1926).

Lindgren, K. M., Douglas, R. C., Couch, R. B.: "Significance of herpesvirus hominis in respiratory secretions of man" *N. Eng. J. Med. 278,* 517, 1968.

Liotet, S., Bonnin, P.: "Diagnostic de l'herpès cornean par immunofluorescence" *Arch. Ophthalmol. 25,* 301, 1965.

Lipschütz, B.: "Untersuchugen über die Ätiologie der Krankheiten der Herpesgruppe (Herpes zoster, Herpes genitalis, Herpes febrilis)" *Arch. Dermatol. Syph. 136,* 428, 1921.

Lipschütz, B.: "Neurodermatrope infektionen (Krankheitein der Herpesgruppe Unna)", in *Handbuch der Haut- und Geschlechts-Krankheiten* (Springer, Berlin, 1923).

Little, J. M., Centifanto, Y. M., Kaufman, H. E.: "Immunoglobulins in human tears" *Am. J. Ophthalmol. 68,* 898, 1969.

London, W. T., Catalano, L. W., Nahmias, A., Fucillo, D. A., Sever, J. L.: "Genital herpes virus hominis type II infection of monkeys" *Obstet. Gynecol. 37,* 501, 1971.

Longson, M., Beswick, T. S. L.: "Dexamethasone treatment in herpes simplex encephalitis" *Lancet 1,* 749, 1971.

Löwenstein, A.: "Aetiologische Untersuchungen über den fieberhafter Herpes" *Münch. Med. Wschr. 66,* 769, 1919.

Lynch, F. W.: "Kaposi's varicelliform eruption" *Arch. Dermatol. Syph. 51,* 129, 1945.

Lynch, F. W., Steves, R. J.: "Kaposi's varicelliform eruption" *Arch. Dermatol. Syph. 55,* 327, 1947.

Lynfield, Y. I., Farhangi, M., Runnels, J. I.: "Generalized herpes simplex complicating lymphoma" *JAMA 207,* 944, 1969.

MacCallum, F. O.: "Generalized herpes simplex in the neonatal period" *Acta Virol. 3,* 17, 1959.

MacCallum, F. O., Juel-Jensen, B. E.: "Herpes simplex virus skin infection in man treated with idoxyuridine in dimethyl sulphoxide: results of double-blind controlled trial" *Brit. Med. J. 2,* 805, 1966.

MacCallum, F. O., Partridge, J. W.: "Fetal-maternal relationship in herpes simplex" *Arch. Dis. Child. 43,* 265, 1968.

MacCallum, F. O., Potter, J. M., Edwards, D. H.: "Early diagnosis of herpes simplex encephalitis by brain biopsy" *Lancet 2,* 322, 1964.

Mao, J. C. H., Robischaw, E., Overby, L. R.: "Inhibition of DNA polymerase from herpes simplex virus-infected Wi-38 cells by phosphonoacetic acid" *J. Virol. 15,* 1281, 1975.

Marinesco, G., Draganesco, S.: "Recherches experimentales sur le neutropisme du virus herpetique" *Ann. Inst. Pasteur, Paris 37,* 753, 1923.

Marks, M. I., Joncas, J. H., Mauer, S. M.: "Fatal hepatitis in siblings: isolation of coxackie virus B5 and herpes simplex virus" *Can. Med. Assoc. J. 102,* 1391, 1970.

Marshall, W. S. J.: "Herpes simplex encephalitis treated with idoxuridine and external decompression" *Lancet 579,* 1967.

Martin, E. C.: "Marital and coital factors in cervical cancer" *Am. J. Public Health 57,* 803, 1967.

156

Martin, M. L., Palmer, E. L., Kissling, R. E.: "Complement-fixing antigens of herpes simplex virus types 1 and 2: reactivity of capsid, envelope and soluble antigens" *Infect. Immun. 5,* 248, 1972.

Martinez, I.: "Relationship of squamous cell carcinoma of the cervix uteri to squamous cell carcinoma of the penis" *Cancer 24,* 777, 1969.

Masu'kawa, T., Garancis, J. C., Rytel, M. W., Mattingly, R. F.: "Herpes genitalis virus isolation from human bladder urine" *Acta Cytol. 16,* 416, 1972.

Maxwell, E.: "Treatment of herpes keratitis with 5-iodo-2-deoxyuridine (IDU). A clinical evaluation of 1500 cases" *Am. J. Ophthalmol. 56,* 571, 1963.

McCormick, D. P.: "Herpes simplex virus as cause of Bell's palsy" *Lancet 1,* 937, 1972.

McCoy, G. A., Leopold, I. H.: "Steroid treatment of herpes simplex infections of the cornea" *Am. J. Ophthalmol. 49,* 1355, 1960.

McDonald, A., Feiwel, M.: "Isolation of herpes virus from erythema multiforme" *Brit. Med. J. 2,* 570, 1970. 257

McDonald, A. D., Williams, M. C., West, R., Stewart, J.: "Neutralizing antibodies to herpes types 1 and 2 in Montreal women" *Am. J. Epidemiol. 100,* 124, 1974 a.

McDonald, A. D., Williams, M. C., Manfreda, J., West, R.: "Neutralizing antibodies to herpesvirus types 1 and 2 in carcinoma of the cervix, carcinoma in situ and cervical dysplasia" *Am. J. Epidemiol. 2,* 130, 1974 b.

McDougal, R. A., Beamer, P. R., Hellerstein, S.: "Fatal herpes simplex hepatitis in a newborn infant" *Am. J. Clin. Pathol. 24,* 1250, 1954.

McKee, A. P.: "Herpes simplex encephalitis" *South. Med. J. 61,* 217, 1968.

McKenzie, D.: "Disseminated herpes simplex infection" *S. Afr. Med. J. 35,* 133, 1961.

McKenzie, D., Hansen, J. D. L., Becker, W.: "Herpes simplex virus infection: dissemination in association with malnutrition" *Arch. Dis. Child. 34,* 250, 1959.

McKelvey, E. M., Kwaan, H. C.: "Cytozine arabinoside therapy for disseminated herpes zoster in a patient with IgG pyroglobulinemia" *Blood 34,* 706, 1969.

Merigan, T. C., Stevens, D. A.: "Viral infections in man associated with acquired immunological deficiency states" *Fed. Proc. 30,* 1858, 1971.

Meyer, J. S., Bauer, R. B., Rivera-Olmos, V. M., Nolan, D. C., Andlerner, A. M.: "Herpes virus hominis encephalitis: neurological manifestations and use of idoxyuridine" *Arch. Neurot. 23,* 438, 1970.

Meyers, R. L., Pettit, T. H.: "Corneal immune response to herpes simplex virus antigens" *J. Immunol. 110,* 1575, 1973.

Middelkamp, J. N., Reed, C. A., Patrizi, G.: "Placental transfer of herpes simplex virus in pregnant rabbits" *Proc. Soc. Exp. Biol. Med. 125,* 757, 1967.

Millar, J. H. D., Haire, M., Fraser, K. B.: "Herpes simplex and temporal lobe epilepsy" *Brit. Med. J. 1,* 471, 1972.

Miller, D., Goldman, J. M., Goldman, M. L.: "Etiologic study of nasopharyngeal cancer" *Arch. Otolaryngol. 94,* 104, 1971.

Miller, D. R., Hanshaw, J. B., O'Leary, D. S., Hnilicka, J. V.: "Fatal disseminated herpes simplex virus infection and hemorrhage in the neonate. Coagulation studies in a case and a review" *J. Pediatr. 76,* 409, 1970.

Miller, J. D., Ross, C. A. C.: "Encephalitis: a four-year survey" *Lancet 1,* 1121, 1968.

Mitchell, J. E., McCallum, F. C.: "Transplacental infection by herpes simplex virus" *Am. J. Dis. Child. 106*, 207, 1963.

Miller, J. K., Hesser, F., Tompkins, V. N.: "Herpes simplex encephalitis: report of 20 cases" *Ann. Intern. Med.* 64, 92, 1966.

Miyamoto, K., Morgan, G., Hsu, K. C., Hampar, B.: "Differentiation by immunoferritin of herpes simplex virion antigens with the use of rabbit 7 S and 19 S antibodies from early (7 day) and late (7 week) immune sera" *J. Natl. Cancer Inst. 46*, 629, 1971.

Moglievska, Z. I.: "Herpetic hepatitis in adults" *Ref. in Ztschr. Mikrobiol. Epidemiol. Immunobiol. 46*, 132, 1969.

Monif, G. R., Brunell, P. A., Hsiung, G. D.: "Visceral involvement by herpes simplex virus in eczema herpeticum" *Am. J. Dis. Child. 116*, 324, 1968.

Montgomerie, J. Z., Becroft, D. M. O., Croxson, M. C., Doah, P. B., North, T. P. K.: "Herpes simplex virus infection after renal transplantation" *Lancet 2*, 867, 1969.

Morgan, H. R., Finland, M.: "Isolation of herpes virus from a case of atypical pneumonia and erythema exudativum multiforme with studies of four additional cases" *Am. J. Med. Sci. 217*, 92, 1949.

Mori, R.: "Effect of neonatal thymectomy on protective immunity of mice against viral infections" *Acta Haematol. Japan 30*, 115, 1967.

Moses, H. L., Cheatham, W. J.: "The frequency and significance of human herpetic esophagitis" *Lab. Invest. 12*, 663, 1963.

Mourriseau, P. M., Phillips, C. A., Leadbetter, G. W.: "Viral prostatitis" *J. Urol. 103*, 767, 1970.

Mozziconacci, P.: "L'herpes nouveau-ne" *Rev. Prat. 11*, 2323, 1961.

Mozziconacci, P., Rivron, J., Habib, R.: "Les hepatites a virus herpetique de nouveau-ne" *Rev. Int. Hepatol. 8*, 1205, 1955.

Muller, S. A., Herrmann, E. C.: "Association of stomatitis and paronychias due to herpes simplex" *Arch. Dermatol. 101*, 396, 1970.

Muller, S. A., Herrmann, E. C., Winkelmann, R. K.: "Herpes simplex infections in hematologic malignancies" *Am. J. Med. 52*, 102, 1972.

Murray, J. O.: "Stevens-Johnson syndrome. Report of two cases" *Lancet 1*, 328, 1947.

Music, S. I., Fine, E. M., Togo, Y.: "Zoster-like disease in the newborn due to herpes simplex" *New Eng. J. Med. 184*, 1, 24, 1971.

Myers, M. G., Oxman, M. N., Clarck, J. E.: "Failure of neutral-red photodynamic inactivation in recurrent herpes simplex virus infections" *New Eng. J. Med., 293*, 945, 1975.

Nahmias, A. J.: "Disseminated herpes simplex virus infection" *New Eng. J. Med. 282*, 684, 1970.

Nahmias, A. J.: "Infections caused by herpesvirus hominis," in Hoeprich, P., ed., pp. 841—852, *Infectious diseases* (Harper and Row, New York, 1972).

Nahmias, A. J., Dowdle, W. R.: "Antigenic and biologic differences in herpesvirus hominis" *Progr. Med. Virol. 10*, 110, 1968.

Nahmias, A. J., Hagler, W. S.: "Ocular manifestations of herpes simplex in the newborn (neonatal ocular herpes)" *Int. Ophthalmol. Clin. 12*, 2, 191, 1972.

Nahmias, A. J., Hutton, R. D.: "Herpes simplex," p. 301—310 in Top, F. H. and Wehrle, P. F., eds., *Communicable and Infectious Diseases* (Mosby, St. Louis, 1972).

158

Nahmias, A. J., Josey, W. E.: "Epidemiology of herpes simplex viruses 1 and 2 in Evans, A. S.: "*Viral Infections of Humans*", (Wiley, New York, 1976,) Ch. 11, p. 253.

Nahmias, A. J., Roizman, B.: "Infections with herpes simplex viruses 1 and 2" *New Eng. J. Med. 667*, 1973.

Nahmias, A. J., Josey, W. E., Naib, Z. M.: "Neonatal herpes simplex infection" *JAMA 199*, 3, 132, 1967a.

Nahmias, A. J., Josey, W. E., Naib, Z. M.: "Neonatal herpes simplex infection: role of genital infection in mother as the source of virus in the newborn" *JAMA 199*, 164, 1967b.

Nahmias, A. J., Naib, Z. M., Highsmith, A., Josey, W. E.: "Experimental genital herpes simplex infection in the mouse" *Pediatr. Res. 1*, 209, 1967c.

Nahmias, A. J., Dowdle, W. R., Naib, Z. M., Josey, W. E., Luce, C. F.: "Genital infection with herpes virus hominis type 1 and 2 in children" *Pediatrics, 42*, 659, 1968.

Nahmias, A. J., Dowdle, W. R., Naib, Z. M., Josey, W. E., McLone, D., Domescik, G.: "Genital infection with type 2 herpes virus hominis" *Brit. J. Vener. Dis. 45*, 294, 1969a.

Nahmias, A. J., Dowdle, W. R., Kramer, J. H., Luce, F. C., Mansour, S. C.: "Antibodies to herpes virus hominis types 1 and 2 in the rabbit" *J. Immunol. 102*, 956, 1969b.

Nahmias, A. J., Dowdle, W. R., Josey, W. E., Naib, Z. M., Painter, L. M., Luce, C.: "Newborn infection with herpes virus hominis type 1 and type 2" *J. Pediatr. 75*, 1194, 1969c.

Nahmias, A. J., Hirsch, S. H., Kramer, H. J., Murphy, F. A.: "Effect of antithymocyte serum on herpesvirus hominis (type 1) infection in adult mice" *Proc. Soc. Exp. Biol. Med. 132*, 696, 1969d.

Nahmias, A. J., Alford, C. A., Korones, S. B.: "Infections of the newborn with herpesvirus hominis" *Adv. Pediatr., 17*, 185, 1970a.

Nahmias, A. L., Josey, W. E., Naib, Z. H., Luce, C. F., Duffey, A.: "Antibodies to herpesvirus hominis type 1 and 2 in humans" *Am. J. Epid. 91*, 539, 1970b.

Nahmias, A. L., Josey, V. E., Naib, Z. M., Luce, C. F., Guest, B. A.: "Antibodies to herpes virus hominis type 1 and 2 in humans. II, Women with cervical cancer" *Am. J. Epid. 91*, 547, 1970c.

Nahmias, A. J., Naib, Z. M., Josey, W. E., Murphy, F. A., Luce, C. F.: "Sarcomas after inoculation of newborn hamsters with herpesvirus hominis type 2 strains" *Proc. Soc. Exp. Biol. Med. 134*, 1065, 1970d.

Nahmias, A. J., Josey, W. E., Naib, Z. M., Freeman, M. G., Fernandez, R. Y., Wheeler, J. H.: "Perinatal risk associated with maternal genital herpes simplex virus infection" *Am. J. Obstet. Gynecol., 110*, 825, 1971a.

Nahmias, A. J., London, W. T., Catalano, L. W.: "Genital herpes virus type 2 infection: an experimental model in Cebus monkeys" *Science 171*, 297, 1971b.

Nahmias, A. J., Wals, K. W., Stewart, J. A., Herrmann, K. Z., Flynt, W. J.: "The TORCH complex: perinatal infections associated with toxoplasma and rubeola, cytomegal and herpes simplex viruses" *Pediatr. Res. 5*, 405, 1971c.

Nahmias, A. J., Ryan, F., Josey, W. E.: "Genital herpes simplex virus infection and gonorrhea: association and analogies" *Brit. J. Vener. Dis. 49*, 306, 1973a.

Nahmias, A. J., Naib, Z. M., Josey, W. E., Franklin, E., Jenkins, R.: "Prospective studies of the association of genital herpes simplex infections and cervical anaplasia" *Cancer Res. 33, 1491,* 1973b.

Nahmias, A. J., Shore, S. L., DelBuono, I in "Viral immunodiagnosis (edited by E. Kurstak and R. Morisset; p. 1965, New York, 1974.

Nahmias, A. J., Josey, W. E., Oleske, J. M.: "Epidemiology of cervical cancer" Ch. 25, p. 501, in Evans, A. S.: *Viral Infections of Humans* Wiley, New York, 1976.

Naib. Z. M.: "Exfoliative cytology of viral cervicovaginitis" *Acta Cytol.* 10, 126, 1966.

Naib, Z. M., Nahmias, A. J., Josey, W. E.: "Cytology and histopathology of cervical herpes simplex infection" *Cancer 19,* 1026, 1966.

Naib, Z. M., Nahmias, A. J., Josey, W. E., Kramer, J. H.: "Genital herpetic infection in association with cervical dysplasia and carcinoma" *Cancer, 23,* 940, 1969.

Naib, Z. M., Nahmias, A. J., Josey, W. E., Wheeler, J. H.: "Association of maternal genital herpetic infection with spontaneous abortion" *Obstet Gynecol. 35,* 260, 1970.

Naib, Z. M., Nahmias, A. J., Josey, W. E., Zaki, S. A.: "Relation of cytohistopathology of genital herpesvirus infection to cervical anaplasia" *Cancer Res. 33,* 1452, 1973.

Nasemann, T.: "Ueber das postherpetische erythema multiforme exudativum" *Hautarzt 15,* 346, 1964.

Nasemann, T., Nagai, R.: "Die Urethritis herpetica: Herpes simplex urethralis" *Münch. Med. Wschr. 102,* 431, 1960.

Nasemann, T. H., Braun-Falco, Q.: "Vinstatische Substanzen in der lokalbehandlung herpetisher Dermatosen" *Therapie Ggw. 109,* 222, 1970.

Nash, G., Foley, F. D.: "Herpetic infection of the middle and lower respiratory tract" *Am. J. Clin. Pathol. 54,* 857, 1970.

Nataf, R., Lepine, P., Bonamour, G.: *Oeil et virus* (Masson, Paris, 1960.).

Neff, J. M., Lane, M. J.: "Vaccinia necrosum following smallpox vaccination for chronic herpetic ulcer" *JAMA 213,* 123, 1970.

Neimann, N., Pierson, M., De Lavergne, E.: "La maladie herpètique du nouveau-né" *Ann. Ped. 10,* 27, 1963. (Sem. Hop. Paris).

Neimann, N., Pierson, M., De Lavergne, E., Gizgengrantz, S., Olive, D.: "La primoinfection herpètique" *Arch. Fr. Pediatr. 3,* 273, 1964.

Nesburn, A. B., Cook, M. L., Stevens, J. G.: "Latent herpes simplex virus isolation from rabbit trigeminal ganglia between episodes of recurrent ocular infection" *Arch. Ophthalmol. 88,* 412, 1972.

Netter, R., Franceschini, P., Chaniot, S.: "Traitement local de 32 malades atteints d'herpès cutanèomuqueux par larifamycine SV ou la rifampicine" *Nouv. Presse. Mèd. 1,* 2403, 1971.

Ng, A. B. P., Reagan, J. W., Lindner, S.: "The cellular manifestations of primary and recurrent herpes genitalis" *Acta Cytol. 14,* 3, 124, 1970a.

Ng, A. B. P., Reagan, J. W., Yen, S. S. L.: "Herpes genitalis. (Clinical and cytopathologic experience with 256 patients)" *Obst. Gynecol. 36,* 645 1970b.

Nicolau, S., Poincloux, P.: "Etude clinique et experimentale d'un cas d'herpès recidivant du doigt" *Ann. Inst. Pasteur. 38,* 977, 1924.

Nigogosyan, G., Mills, J.: "Herpes simplex cervicitis" *JAMA 191,* 496, 1965.

Nishimura, K., Nagamoto, A., Igarashi, M.: "Extensive skin manifestations of herpesvirus infection in an acute leukemic child" *Pediatrics 49*, 294, 1972.

Nishimura, L.: "Antigenic relation of S. M. O. N. associated virus to herpesvirus group" *Lancet 1*, 159, 1973.

Nolan, D. C., Carruthers, M. M., Lerner, A. M.: "Herpes virus hominis encephalitis in Michigan: report of thirteen cases, including six treated with idoxyuridine" *New Eng. J. Med. 282*, 10, 1970.

Nolan, D. C., Lauter, C. B., Lerner, A. M.: "Idoxyuridine in Herpes simplex virus (type 1) encephalitis" *Ann. Intern. Med. 78*, 243, 1973.

Notkins, A. L., Mergenhagen, S. E., Howard, J. R.: "Effect of virus infections on the function of the immune system" *Ann. Rev. Microbiol. 24*, 525, 1970.

Nuget, G. R., Chou, S. M.: "Treatment of labial herpes" *JAMA 224*, 132, 1973.

Offret, G., Douliquen, Y., Camp. C.: "L'homogreffe de la cornee dans la keratitis herpètique" *Arch. Ophthalmol. 26*, 561, 1966.

Okada, Y., Kim, J.: "Interaction of concanavalin A with enveloped viruses and host cells" *Virology 50*, 507, 1972.

Olshevsky, V., Becker, Y.: "Herpes simplex virus structural protein" *Virology 40*, 948, 1970.

Olson, L., Beuscher, E. L., Artenstein, M. S., Parkman, P. D.: "Herpes virus infections of the central nervous system" *New Eng. J. Med. 277*, 1271, 1967.

O'Neill, F. I., Rapp, F.: "Synergistic effect of herpes simplex virus and cytosine arabinoside on human chromosomes" *J. Virol. 7*, 692, 1971.

Orkin, F. K.: "Herpetic whitlow" *New Eng. J. Med. 292*, 648, 1975.

Ortona, L., Pizzigallo, E., Gelfo, P.: "Studio sugli anticorpi fissanti il complemento contro il virus dell'herpes simplex e dell'herpes varicellae-zoster. Rapporti con i sindromi neurologische ad eziologia ignota" *Giorn. Mal. Inf. Par. 24*, 11, 813, 1972.

Overall, J. C., Glasow, L. A.: "Virus infections of the fetus and newborn infant" *J. Pediatr. 77*, 315, 1970.

Oxbury, J. M., McCallum, F. O.: "Herpes simplex encephalitis" *Postgrad. Med. J. 49*, 383, 1973.

Page, L. K., Tyler, H. R., Shillite, J.: "Neurosurgical experiences with herpes simplex encephalitis" *J. Neurosurg. 27*, 346, 1967.

Paine, T. F.: "Herpetic meningo-encephalitis" *Bacteriol. Rev. 28*, 372, 1964.

Pandi, D. N.: "Herpetic erythema multiforme" *Brit. Med. J. 1*, 746, 1964.

Panijel, J., Cayeux, P.: "Immunosuppressive effects of macrophage antiserum" *Immunology 14*, 769, 1968.

Park, J. H., Baron, S.: "Herpetic keratoconjunctivitis: therapy with synthetic double stranded RNA" *Science 162*, 811, 1968.

Park, J. H., Galin, M. A., Billau, A., Baron, S.: "Prophylaxis of herpetic keratoconjunctivitis with interferon inducers" *Arch. Ophthalmol. 81*, 840, 1969.

Parker, J. D. J., Banatvala, J. E.: "Herpes genitalis. Clinical and virological studies" *Brit. J. Vener. Dis. 43*, 212, 1967.

Partridge, J. W., Millis, R. R.: "Systemic herpes simplex infection in a newborn treated intravenous idoxyuridine" *Arch. Dis. Child. 43*, 377, 1968.

Paschetta, G.: "Realazione sull'attività della distamycima A (F. I. 6426) farmaco antivirale" *Giorn. Mal. Inf. Paras. 24*, 795, 1972.

Pasricha, J. S., Nayyar, K. C., Pasricha, A.: "A new method for treatment of herpes simplex" *Arch. Dermatol. 107*, 775, 1973.

Patrizi, G., Middelkamp, J. N., Read, C. A.: "Fine structure of herpes simplex virus and hepatoadrenal necrosis in the newborn" *Am. J. Clin. Pathol. 49*, 325, 1968.

Pavan-Langston, D., Dohlman, C. H.: "Double-blind clinical study of adenine arabinoside therapy of viral keratoconjunctivitis" *Am. J. Ophthalmol. 74*, 81, 1972.

Pavan-Langston, D., McCulley, J. P.: "Herpes zoster dendritic keratitis" *Arch. Ophthalmol. 89*, 25, 1973.

Perol, Y., Laufer, M. J.: "Stomatite herpetique de primoinfection chez un adolescent, compliquée de quatre perionyxis de meme étiologie" *Bull. Soc. Fr. Derm. Syph. 74*, 421, 1967.

Person, D. A., Sheridan, P. J., Herrmann, E. C.: "Sensitivity of types 1 and 2 herpes virus to 5-iodo-2-deoxyuridine and 9-beta-D-arabino furanosyladenine" *Infect. Immun. 2*, 815, 1970.

Person, D. A., Kaufman, R. H., Gardner, H. L., Rawls, W. E.: "Herpes virus type 2 in genitourinary tract infections" *Am. J. Obstet. Gynecol. 116*, 993, 1973.

Pettay, O., Leinikki, P., Donner, L., Lapinleimu, K.: "Herpes simplex infection of the newborn" *Arch. Dis. Child. 47*, 97, 1972.

Pien, F. D., Smith, T. F., Anderson, C. F.: "Herpesvirus in renal transplant patients" *Transplant 16*, 5, 489, 1973.

Pierce, N. F., Portnoy, B., Leeds, N. E., Morrison, R. L., Wehrle, P.: "Encephalitis associated with herpes simplex infection presenting as a temporal-lobe mass: report of two cases with survival" *Neurol. survival 14*, 708, 1964.

Piringer, W.: "Epidemisches Auftreten von Herpes simplex" *Klin. Med. 13*, 533, 1958.

Plummer, G.: "Comparative virology of the herpes group" *Progr. Med. Virol., 9*, 302, 1967.

Plummer, G.: "A review of the identification and titration of antibodies to herpes simplex viruses type 1 and type 2 in human sera" *Cancer Res. 33*, 1469, 1973.

Plummer, G., Hackett, S.: "Herpes simplex virus and paralysis of animals" *Brit. J. Exp. Pathol. 47*, 82, 1966.

Plummer, G., Masterson, J. G.: "Herpes simplex and cancer of the cervix" *Am. J. Obstet. Gynecol. 3*, 81, 1971.

Plummer, G., Waner, J. L., Bowling, C. P.: "Comparative studies of type 1 and 2 herpes simplex viruses" *Brit. J. Exp. Pathol. 49*, 202, 1968.

Plummer, G., Waner, J. L., Phuangsab, A., Goodheart, C. R.: "Type 1 and 2 herpes simplex viruses: serological and biological differences" *J. Virol. 5*, 51, 1970.

Pollikoff, P., Cannavale, P., Di Puppo, A.: "Effect of complexed synthetic RNA analogues on herpes simplex virus infection in rabbit cornea" *Am. J. Ophthalmol. 69*, 650, 1970.

Pollikoff, T.: "Topical vaccine therapy in herpetic keratitis" *Lancet 1*, 1064, 1970.

162

Poluiquen, Y., Jollivet, J., Argenton, C.: "Code d'utilisation du vaccin anti-herpètique en pratique ophthalmologique" *Arch. Ophthalmol. 26*, 565, 1966.

Porter, D. D., Wimbery, J., Bengemh-Melnick, M.: "Prevalence of anti-bodies to EB virus and other herpesviruses" *JAMA 208*, 1675, 1969.

Porter, P. S., Baughman, R. D.: "Epidemiology of herpes simplex among wrestlers" *JAMA 194*, 998, 1965.

Poste, G., King, N.: "Isolation of herpes virus from the canine genital tract: association with infertility, abortion and stillbirths" *Vet. Res., 88*, 229, 1971.

Poste, G., Hawkins, D. F., Thomlinson, J.: "Herpesvirus hominis infection of the female genital tract" *Obstet. Gynecol. 40*, 6, 871, 1972.

Price, R., Chernik, N. L., Horta-Barbosa, L., Posner, J. B.: "Herpes simplex encephalitis in an anergic patient" *Am. J. Med. 54*, 222, 1973.

Priden, J., Lilienfeld, A. M.: "Carcinoma of the cervix in Jewish women in Israel 1960, 1967. An epidemiological survey" *Israeli J. Med. Sci. 7*, 1465, 1971.

Proto, F., Tedesco, N.: "Osservazioni su di un caso di cheratite erpetica neonatale" *Boll. Ocul. 45*, 573, 1966.

Prusoff, W. H., Goz, B.: "Chemotherapy molecular aspects pp. 642—660," in Kaplan, A. S. ed., *The herpesviruses* (Academic Press, New York, 1973).

Pugh, R. C. B., Newns, G. H., Dudgeon, J. A.: "Hepatic necrosis in disseminated herpes simplex" *Arch. Dis. Child. 29*, 60, 1954.

Pugh, R. C. B., Dudgeon, J. A., Bodian, M. J.: "Kaposi's varicelliform eruption (eczema herpeticum) with typical and atypical visceral necrosis" *J. Path. Bact. 69*, 67, 1955.

Quilligan, J. J., Wilson, J. L.: "Fatal herpes simplex infection in a newborn infant" *J. Lab. Clin. Med. 38*, 742, 1951.

Rabson, A.: "Herpesvirus and cancer: introduction" *Fed. Proc. 31*, 6, 1625, 1972.

Rada, B., Altanerova, V.: "Virus inhibition activity of 6-azauridine dependent on cell-free extracts containing uridine kinase. I, Inhibition of plaque-formation" *Acta Virol. 14*, 425, 1970.

Rada, B., Hanušovska, T.: "Virus-inhibitory activity of 6-azauridine dependent on cell-free extracts containing uridine kinase. II, Quantitative aspects, efficacy of pretreatment" *Acta Virol. 14*, 435, 1970.

Radcliffe, W. B., Guinto, F. C., Adcock, D. G., Krigman, M. R.: "Herpes simplex encephalitis: a radiologic study of four cases" *New Eng. J. Med. 112*, 263, 1971.

Ragazzini, F.: "Considerazioni su di un grave quadro recidivante da virus dell'-herpes simplex in corso di meningoencephalite tubercolare" *Giorn. Mal. Inf. Par. 14*, 692, 1962.

Rapp, F., Duff, R.: "In vitro cell transformation by herpesviruses" *Fed. Proc. 31*, 6, 1660, 1972.

Rapp, F., Duff, R.: "Transformation of hamster embryo fribroblasts by herpes simplex viruses type 1 and 2" *Cancer Res. 33*, 1527, 1973.

Rapp, F., Jui-Lien, H. L., Jerkofsky, M.: "Transformation of mammalian cells by DNA-containing viruses following photodynamic inactivation" *Virology 55*, 339, 1973.

Rappel, M.: "Treatment of herpes encephalitis" *Lancet 1*, 971, 1971.

Rappel, M., Dubois-Dalcq, M., Sprecher, S., Thiry, L., Lowenthal, A., Pelc, S., Thys, J. P.: "Diagnosis and treatment of herpes encephalitis. A multi-disciplinary approach" *J. Neurol. Sci. 12*, 443, 1971.

Rasmussen, L. E., Jordan, G. W., Stevens, D. A., Merigan, T. C.: "Lymphocyte interferon production and transformation after herpes simplex infection in humans" *J. Immunol. 112*, 728, 1974.

Ravaut, P., Darre, R.: "Les reactions nerveuses au cour des herpes genitaux" *Ann. Dermat. Syph. 5*, 481, 1904.

Rawls, W. E.: "Encephalitis associated with herpes simplex virus" *Ann. Intern. Med. 64*, 104, 1966.

Rawls, W. E.: "Herpes simplex virus" pp. in Kaplan, A. S. ed., *The Herpesviruses* (Academic Press, New York, 1973).

Rawls, W. E., Laurel, D., Melnick, J. L., Glicman, J. M., Kaufman, R. J.: "A search for viruses in smegma, premalignant and early malignant cervical tissues. The isolation of herpes viruses with distinct carcinogenic properties" *Am. J. Epidemiol., 87*, 3, 1968a.

Rawls, W. E., Tompkins, W. A. F., Fihueroa, M. E., Melnick, J. L.: "Herpes virus type 2: association with carcinoma of the cervix" *Science 161*, 1255, 1968b.

Rawls, W. E., Tompkins, W. A. F., Melnick, L.: "The association of herpesvirus type 2 and carcinoma of the uterine cervix" *Am. J. Epidemiol. 89* 5547, 1969.

Rawls, W. E., Gardner, H. L., Kaufman, R. L.: "Antibodies to genital herpesvirus in patients with carcinoma of the cervix" *Am. Obstet. Gynecol. 107*, 5, 710, 1970a.

Rawls, W. E., Iwamoto, K., Adam, E., Melnick, J. K.: "Measurement of antibodies to herpesvirus types 1 and 2 in human sera" *J. Immunol. 104*, 599, 1970b.

Rawls, W. E., Gardner, H. L., Flanders, E. W., Lowry, S. P., Kaufman, R. H., Melnick, J. L.: "Genital herpes in two social groups" *Am. J. Gynecol. 110*, 682, 1971.

Rawls, W. E., Adam, E., Melnick, J.: "An analysis of seroepidemiological studies of herpesvirus type 2 and carcinoma of the cervix" *Cancer Res. 33*, 1477, 1973.

Ray, E. K., Halpern, B. L., Levitan, D. B., Blough, H. A.: "A new approach to viral chemotherapy. Inhibitors of glycoprotein synthesis" *Lancet 2*, 680, 1974.

Reed, J. A., Sever, J., Kurtzke, J.: "Measles antibody in patients with multiple sclerosis" *Arch. Neurol. 10*, 402, 1964.

Rekant, S. I.: "Eczema herpeticum and pregnancy" *Obstet. Gynecol. 31*, 387, 1973.

Rendtorf, R. C., Fowinkle, E. W.: "Herpes simplex skin lesions simulating smallpox" *JAMA 192*, 156, 1965.

Ribarić, V.: "*Ispitivanje djelovanja Bimolina na herpetični keratitis laboratorijskih životinja*" Magisterski rad (Effects of Bimolin on Herpetic Keratitis of Laboratory Animals) (master's thesis), Rijeka, 1968.

Ribarić, V.: "Lokalna terapija herpetičnog keratitisa zamoraca Bimolinom" (Local therapy of herpetic keratitis in guinea pigs using Bimolin) *Saopćenja (Pliva, Zagreb) 2*, 55, 1970.

164

Ribarić, V.: "Mehanizam terapijskog djelovanja kriopeksije kod herpetičnog keratitisa" (Mechanism of therapeutic action of cryopexia in herpetic keratitis) *Liječ. Vjesn. 95*, 207, 1973.

Ribarić, V.: "Opća piretoterapija herpetičnog keratitisa zamoraca" (General pyretic therapy of herpetic keratitis in guinea pigs) *Medica Jadertina 1—2*, 59, 1974.

Ribarić, V.: "Teorija dualiteta osjeta rožnice kod herpetičnog keratitisa" (Theory of sensory dualily of the carnea in herpetic keratitis) *Jug. Oftal. Arhiv 1/2*, 49, 1974.

Ribarić, V.: "Koncentracija plazmotskih i urinarnih kateholamina kod herpetičnog keratitisa; tonus simpatikusa" (Concentration of plasmatic and urninary catecholamines in herpetic keratitis) in Proceedings of the 5th European Ophthalmological Congress, Hamburg, 1976.

Ribarić, V.: „Klasifikacija herpetičnog keratitisa" (Classification of herpetic keratitis) 1976. (to be published)

Ribarić, V., Batistić, B.: "Slučaj letalnog herpesa virusa encefalitisa zamorca" (Fatal herpesvirus encephalitis in a guinea pig) *Acta Ophthalmol. Jug. 3*, 226, 1973.

Ribarić, V., Gligo, D.: "Efekat različitih terapeutskih metoda kod herpetičnog keratitisa" (Efficacy of different methods of treating herpetic keratitis) *Acta Ophthalmol. Jug. 1/2*, 40, 1972.

Ribarić, V., Batistić, B., Gligo, D.: "Patohistološke promjene rožnice čovjeka kod kriopeksije rožnice" (Pathohistological changes after cryopexia of the human carnea) *Acta Fac. Med. Fluminensis 1/2*, 211, 1971/72.

Richardson, J., Crombie, A. L., Gardner, P. S., McQuillin, J.: "Diagnosis of herpesvirus hominis keratitis by immunofluorescence" *Brit. J. Ophthalmol. 53*, 616, 1969.

Rimon, R., Halonen, P.: cit. by (Leobury *et al. Dis. Nerv. Syst. 30*, 338, 1969)

Robinskon, T. W. E., Dover, J. R.: "Experimental zosteriform herpes simplex virus infection in mouse skin" *Brit. J. Dermatol. 86*, 40, 1972.

Robinson, M. G., Kauffman, S.: "Disseminated herpes simplex: a cause of consumption coagulopathy" *Soc. Pediatr. Res. Abst. 103*, 1969.

Roizman, B., Frenkel, N.: "The transcription and state of herpes simplex virus DNA in productive infection and in human cervical cancer tissue" *Cancer Res. 33*, 1402, 1973.

Roizman, B., Keller, J. M., Spear, P. G., Terni, M., Nahmias, A. J., Dowdle, W.: "Variability of structural glycoproteins and classification of herpes simplex viruses" *Nature 227*, 1253, 1970.

Rook, A.: "Association of erythema multiforme with herpes simplex" *Brit. Med. J. 1*, 328, 1947.

Rosato, E. F., Rosato, M., Plotkin, S. A.: "Herpetic paronychia: an occupational hazard of medical personnel" *New Eng. J. Med. 804*, 1970.

Rose, A. G., Becker, W. B.: "Disseminated herpesvirus hominis (herpes simplex) infection: retrospective diagnosis by light and electron microscopy of paraffin max-embedded tissues" *J. Clin. Pathol. 25*, 79, 1972.

Rosenberg, G. L., Notkins, A. L.: "Induction of cellular immunity to herpes simplex virus: relationship to the humoral immune response" *J. Immunol. 112*, 1019, 1974.

Rosenberg, G. L., Farber, P. A., Notkins, A. L.: "In vitro stimulation of sensitized lymphocytes by herpes simplex virus and vaccinia virus" *Proc. Natl. Acad. Sci. USA 69*, 756, 1972.

Ross, C. A. C., Stevenson, J.: "Herpes simplex meningoencephalitis" *Lancet* *2*, 682, 1961.

Ross, C. A., Lenman, J. A., Rutter, C.: "Infective agents and multiple sclerosis" *Brit. Med. J. 1*, 226, 1965.

Ross, C. A., Lenman, J. A., Melville, I. D.: "Virus antibody levels in multiple sclerosis" *Brit. Med. J. 3*, 512, 1969.

Rotkin, I. D.: "Sexual characteristics of a cervical cancer population" *Amer. J. Publ. Health 57*, 815, 1967.

Rotkin, I. D.: "A comparison review of key epidemiological studies in cervical cancer related to current searches for transmissible agents" *Cancer Res. 33*, 1353, 1973.

Royston, I., Aurelian, L.: "The association of genital herpes viruses with cervical atypia and carcinoma in situ" *Am. J. Epidemiol. 91*, 531, 1970.

Ruchman, I., Dodd, K.: "Kaposi's varicelliform eruption: a primary infection with herpes simplex virus" *Pediatrics 1*, 364, 1948.

Ruiter, M.: "Aphthous stomatitis and herpetic paronychia in an adult" *Acta Dermatovener. 30*, 497, 1950.

Russell, A. S.: "Cell-mediated immunity to herpes simplex virus in man" *J. Infect. Dis. 129*, 142, 1974.

Ryden, F. W., Moses, H. L., Garrote, C. E., Beaver, D. L.: "Herpetic (inclusion-body) encephalitis" *South. Med. J. 58*, 903, 1965.

Sabin, A.: "Misery of recurrent herpes: what to do?" *N. Engl. J. Med. 986*, 1975.

St. Geme, J. W. S., Prince, J. T., Burke, B. A., Good, R. A., Krivitt, W.: "Impaired cellular resistance of herpes simplex virus in Wiscott-Aldrich syndrome" *New Eng. J. Med. 273*, 229, 1965.

Sanders, D. Y., Cramblett, H. G.: "Viral infections in hospitalized neonates" *Am. J. Dis. Child. 116*, 251, 1968.

Santoianni, P.: "La nostra esperienza sulla terapia dell' erpete semplice recidivante con un vaccino specifico" *Minerva Pediatr. 41*, 30, 1966.

Saraux, H.: "La keratite discriforme n'est-elle qu'une allergie virale?" *Arch. Ophthalmol. 26*, 557, 1966.

Sawanobori, S.: "Seroepidemiological study of herpes simplex virus infection. II, Age distribution of neutralizing antibody to herpes simplex virus type I and type II" *Acta Paediatr. Japan 15*, 2, 16, 1973.

Sawanobori, S., Onishi, S., Matsujama, S., Irie, H.: "HSV — I and acute aseptic meningitis" *Lancet II*, 756, 1974.

Scalise, G., Barca, L., Mura, S., Sinicco, A.: "Rilievi sul comportamento delle immunoglobuline del siero e del secreto lacrimale in corso di cheratite da herpes simplex" *Boll. d'Ocul. 50*, 569, 1970.

Scalise, G., Sinico, A., Barca, L.: "Le immunoglobuline del siero e del secreto lacrimalo nella cheratite erpetica" *Giorn. Mal. Infet. Paras. 24*, 817, 1972.

Schaffer, A. J., Avery, M. E.: *Diseases of the Newborn* (Saunders, Philadelphia, 1965).

Schneweis, K. E.: "Serologische Untersuchungen zur Typendifferenzierung des Herpes virus hominis" *Z. Immunitätsforsch. 124*, 24, 1962.

Schofield, C. B. S.: "The treatment of herpes genitalis with S 1000-2-deoxyuridine" *Brit. J. Dermatol. 76*, 465, 1964.

166

Schwartz, R. S.: "Fatal HVH pneumonia in transplant patients treated with ALS" *Hosp. Pract.* 4, 42, 1969.

Scott, T. F. M.: "Infection with the virus herpes simplex" *New Eng. J. Med.* 250, 183, 1954.

Scott, T. F. M.: "Epidemiology of herpetic infection" *Am. J. Ophthalmol.* 43, 134, 1957.

Scott, T. F. M., Prior, P. F.: "The EEG in herpes simplex encephalitis" *Lancet* 2, 525, 1970.

Scott, T. F. M., Tokumaru, T.: "Herpes virus hominis (virus of herpes simplex)" *Bacteriol. Rev.* 28, 458, 1964.

Scott, T. F. M., Tokumaru, T.: "The herpesvirus group," in Horsfall, F. L., and Tamm, I., eds., *Viral and rickettsial infections of man* (Vuk Karadžić, Beograd, 1970).

Scott, T. F. M., Steigman, A. J., Convey, J. H.: "Acute infectious gingivostomatitis: etiology, epidemiology and clinical picture of a common disorder caused by the virus of herpes simplex" *JAMA 117*, 999, 1941.

Scott, T. F. M., Coriell, L. L., Blank, H.: "Infections with the virus of herpes simplex" *Am. J. Dis. Child.*, 79, 951, 1950.

Scott, T. F. M., Coriell, L. L., Blank, H., Burgeon, C. F.: "Some comments on herpetic infection in children with special emphasis on unusual clinical manifestations" *J. Pediatr.* 41, 835, 1952.

Segal, N., Takess, M., Mate, I.: "Crioterapia in tratamentul keratitei herpetice" *Ophtalmologia (Buc.) 11*, 49, 1967.

Seidenberg, S.: "Zur Aetiologie der Pustulosis vacciniformis acuta" *Schweiz Ztschr. Path. u Bakt.* 4, 389, 1941.

Selling, B., Kibrick, S.: "An outbreak of herpes simplex among wrestlers (herpes gladiatorum)" *New Eng. J. Med.* 270, 979, 1964.

Sever, J., White, L. R.: "Intrauterine viral infections" *Ann. Rev. Med.* 19, 471, 1968.

Sexton, R. R.: "Eyelids, lacrimal apparatus and conjunctiva" *Arch. Ophthalmol.* 83, 361, 1970.

Shardein, J. L., Sidwell, R. W.: "Antiviral activity of 9-beta-D-arabinofuranosyzadenine" *Antimicrob. Agent. Chemother. 155*, 1968.

Sharlit, H.: "Herpes progenitalis as a venereal contagion" *Arch. Dermatol.* 43, 933, 1940.

Shelley, W. B.: "Herpes simplex virus as a cause of erythema multiforme" *JAMA 201*, 153, 1967.

Sherman, F. E., Davis, R. L., Haymaker, W.: "Subacute inclusion encephalitis: report of a case with observations on the fluorescent antiherpes simplex antibody reactions" *Acta Neuropathol.* 1, 271, 1961.

Shershow, L. W., Ekert, H., Swansen, V. L., Wright, H. T., Gilerhirst, G. D.: "Intravascular coagulation in generalised herpes simplex infection of the newborn" *Acta Paediatr. Scand.* 58, 535, 1969.

Sheward, J. D.: "Perianal herpes simplex" *Lancet 1*, 315, 1961.

Shin, H., Snyserman, R., Friedman, E., Mellors, A., Mayer, M.: "Chemotactic and anaphylatoxic fragment cleaved from the fifth component of guinea pig complement" *Science 162*, 361, 1968.

Shipkowitz, N. L., Bower, R. R., Appel, R. N.: "Suppression of herpes simplex virus infection by phosphonoacetic acid" *Appl. Microbiol. 26*, 264, 1973.

167

Shubladze, A. K., Chzhu-Shan, K.: "Study on the antigenic properties of herpes virus" *Vopr. Virusol. 4,* 80, 1959.

Sidwell, R. W., Dixon, F. M., Schabel, F. M., Kaump, D. H.: "Antiviral activity of 9-beta-D-arabino furanosyladenine" *Antimicrob. Agent. Chemother. 148,* 1968.

Sieber, F., Fulginiti, V. A., Brazie, J., Umlauf, H. H.: "In utero infection of the fetus by herpes simplex virus" *J. Pediatr. 69,* 30, 1966.

Siegel, I. M.: "Herpetic sciatica" *Surgery 66,* 4, 693, 1969.

Silk, B. R., Roome, A. P. C. H.: "Herpes encephalitis treated with intravenous idoxyuridine" *Lancet 411,* ii, 1970.

Silverstein, E. H., Burnett, J. W.: "Kaposi's varicelliform eruption complication pemphigus foliaceus" *Arch. Dermatol. 95,* 1967.

Simpson, J. R.: "Kaposi's varicelliform eruption: direct transmision to a nurse" *Brit. J. Dermatol. 65,* 139, 1953.

Singer, A.: "Genital herpes and cervical cancer" *Brit. Med. J. 1,* 458, 1971.

Skinner, G. R. B., Thouless, M. E., Jordan, J. A.: "Antibodies to type 1 and type 2 herpes virus in women with abnormal cervical cytology" *J. Obstet. Gynecol. Brit. Commonwealth 78,* 1031, 1971.

Skoldenberg, M.: "On the role of viruses in acute infectious diseases of the central nervous system" *Scand. J. Inf. Dis. Suppl. 3,* 1, 1972.

Slavin, H. B., Gavett, E.: "Primary herpetic vulvovaginitis" *Proc. Soc. Exp. Biol. Med. 63,* 343, 1946.

Slavin, H. Z., Ferguson, J. J.: "Zoster-like eruptions caused by the virus of herpes simplex" *Am. J. Med. 8,* 456, 1950.

Sloan, B. J.: "Treatment of herpes simplex virus type 1 and 2 encephalitis in mice with 9-beta-D-arabino-furanosyladenine" *Antimicrob. Agent. Chemother. 31,* 74, 1973.

Smith, J. W., Peutherer, J. F., McCallum, F. O.: "The incidence of herpesvirus hominis antibody in the population" *J. Hyg. 65,* 395, 1967.

Smith, J. W., Adam, E., Melnick, J. L., Rawls, W. E.: "Use of the 51 Cr release test to demonstrate patterns of antibody response in humans to herpes virus types 1 and 2" *J. Immunol. 109,* 554, 1972a.

Smith, J. W., Lowry, S. D., Melnick, J. L., Rawls, W. E.: "Antibodies to surface antigens of herpesvirus type 1 and type 2 infected cells among women with cervical cancer and control women" *Inf. Immunol. 5,* 305, 1972b.

Smith, M. G., Lennette, F. H., Reames, H. R.: "Isolation of the virus of the herpes simplex and the demonstration of intranuclear inclusions in a case of acute encephalitis" *Am. J. Pathol. 17,* 55, 1941.

Smythe, P. M., Schonland, M., Brereton-Stiles, G. G., Goovadia, H. M., Grace, H. J.: "Thymolymphatic deficiency and depression of cell-mediated immunity in protein-calorie malnutrition" *Lancet 2,* 939, 1971.

Solomon, M.: "Herpes simplex virus from skin lesions of myelogenous leukemia" *Arch. Int. Med. 107,* 168, 1961.

Söltz-Szötz, J.: "Nachweis des Herpes simplex Virus aus Effloreszenzen eines Falles des Erythema exudativum multiforme" *Arch. Haut. Geschl. 34,* 25, 1963.

Söltz-Szötz, J., Fanta, D.: "Viruserkrankungen der Haut" *Hautarzt. 55,* 267, 1974.

Sorice, F.: "La malattia erpetica" *Giorn. Mal. Inf. Paras. 23,* 469, 1971.

168

South, M. A., Tompkins, W. A. F., Morris, R., Rawls, W. E.: "Congenital malformation of the central nervous system associated with genital type 2 herpes virus" *J. Pediatr. 75*, 13, 1969.

Spence, J., Miller, F. W., Court, D.: *Thousand Family Survey — Newcastle, England*, (Oxford University Press, London, 1954).

Spencer, E. S., Anderson, H. K.: "Clinically evident, nonterminal infections with herpesviruses and the wart virus in immunosuppressed renal allograft recipients" *Brit. Med. J. 2*, 251, 1970.

Sprecher-Goldberger, S., Thiry, L., Cattoor, J. P.: "Herpes virus type 2 infection and carcinoma of the cervix" *Lancet 2*, 266, 1970.

Stadler, H., Exman, M. N., Dawson, D. M., Levin, J. M.: "Herpes simplex meningitis: Isolation of herpes simplex virus type 2 from cerebrospinal fluid" *New Eng. J. Med. 1296*, 1973.

Stanković, I., Dučić-Petrović, M.: "Virusni keratitis dječjeg doba" (Viral keratitis in children) *Acta Ophthalmol Iug 3*, 301, 1964.

Stein, P. J., Siciliano, A.: "Necrotizing herpes simplex virus viral infections of the cervix during pregnancy" *Am. J. Obstet. Gynecol. 94*, 249, 1966.

Stern, E., Longo, L. D.: "Identification of herpes simplex virus in a case showing cytological features of viral vaginitis" *Acta Cytol. 1*, 7, 295, 1963.

Stern, H., Elek, S. D., Millar, D. M., Anderson, H. F.: "Herpetic whitlow a form of cross-infection in hospitals" *Lancet 2*, 871, 1959.

Stevens, D. A., Pincus, T., Burroughs, M. A. K., Hampar, B.: "Serologic relationship of a simian herpes virus (SA 8) and herpes simplex virus: heterogeneity in the degree of reciprocal crossreactivity shown by rabbit 7 S and 19 S antibody" *J. Immunol. 101*, 979, 1968.

Stevens, J. G., Cook, M. L.: "Latent herpes simplex virus in spinal ganglia of mice" *Science 173*, 843, 1971.

Stevens, J. G., Nesburn, A. B., Cook, M. L.: "Latent herpes simplex virus from trigeminal ganglia of rabbits with recurrent eye infection" *Nature New. Biol. 235*, 216, 1972.

Stock, E. L., Aronson, S. B.: "Corneal immune globulin distribution" *Arch. Pathol. 84*, 355, 1970.

Ström, J.: "Herpes simplex virus as a cause of allergic mucocutaneous reaction (ectodermosis erosiva pluriorifidalis, Stevens-Johnson syndrome etc.) and general infection" *Scand. J. Inf. Dis. 1*, 3, 1969.

Stroud, M. G.: "Recurrent herpes simplex and steroid dosage in a patient with the nephrotic syndrome due to primary systemic amyloidosis" *Arch. Dermatol. 84*, 396, 1961.

Sutton, A. L., Smithwick, E. M., Seligman, S. J., Kim, D. S.: "Fatal disseminated herpes virus hominis type 2 infection in an adult with associated thymic dysplasia" *Am. J. Med. 56*, 545, 1974.

Švara, V., Božinović, D., Sekula, I., Šćetinec, N.: "Novija saznanja o infekcijama uzrokovanim herpes simplex virusom" (Recent advances in the knowledge of herpes simplex virus infections) *Arhiv ZMD 3*, 211, 1974.

Swyers, J. S., Lausch, R. N., Kaufman, H. E.: "Corneal hypersensitivity to herpes simplex" *Brit. J. Ophthalmol. 51*, 843, 1967.

Szogi, S., Berge, T.: "Generalised herpes simplex in newborns" *Acta Pathol. Microbiol. Scand. 66*, 401, 1966.

Talanyi-Pfeifer, I.: "Prilog liječenju herpetičnog keratitisa Joddesoxiuridinom" (Treatment of herpetic keratitis with iodoxyuridine) *Acta. Ophthalmol. Iug. 1/2*, 48, 1972.

Tamalet, E.: "Meningite herpetique recidivante (17 atteintes en 14 ans)" *Toulouse Med. 36*, 262, 1935.

Tamm, I., "Symposium on the experimental pharmacology and clinical use of antimetabolites. III. Metabolic antagonists and selective virus inhibition" *Clin. Pharmacol. Ther. 1*, 777, 1960.

Tanaka, S., Southam, C. M.: "Zoster-like lesions form herpes simplex virus in newborn rats" *Proc. Soc. Exp. Biol. Med. 120*, 56, 1965.

Teague, O., Goodpasture, E. W.: "Experimental herpes zoster" *J. Med. Res. 44*, 185, 1923 (cit. Slavin. Ana Ferguson, 1950).

Templeton, A. C.: "Generalized HS in malnourished children" *J. Clin. Pathol. 23*, 24, 1970.

Terni, M., Luzzatto, A.: "Virus dell'herpes simplex e sclerosi a plache: indagini virologiche e sierologiche" *Riv. Patol. Nevr. Ment. 90*, 113, 1969.

Terni, M., Caccialanza, P., Cassai, E., Kieff, E.: "Aseptic meningitis in association with herpes progenitalis" *New Eng. J. Med. 1971.*

Thieffry, S., Martin, C., Drouhet, V., Bouchard, J.: "Encephalite herpetique curable. Etude virologique et immunologique" *Arch. Fr. Pediatr. 12*, 573, 1955.

Thygeson, P.: "Chronic herpetic keratouveitis" *Tr. Am. Ophthal. Soc. 65*, 211, 1967.

Thygeson, P., Kimura, S. J.: "Deep forms of herpetic keratitis" *Am. J. Ophthal. 43*, 109, 1957.

Tokumaru, T.: "The protective effects of different immunoglobulins and skin infection in guinea pigs" *Arch. Ges. Virusforsch. 22*, 332, 1968.

Tolentino, P., DeMatteis, F.: "Primo-infezione herpetica con epatite a inclusioni nucleare (rilievo biopsico) in bambino di 4 anni" *Clin. Pediatr. Bologna 35*, 461, 1953.

Tomlinson, A. H., McCallum, F. O.: "The effect of 5-iodo-2-deoxyuridine on herpes simplex virus infections in guinea pig skin" *Brit. J. Exper. Pathol. 49*, 277, 1968.

Tommila, V.: "Treatment of dendritic keratitis with interferon" *Acta Ophthal. 41*, 478, 1963.

Torphy, D. E., Ray, C. G., McAlister, R., Du, J. N. H.: "Herpes simplex virus infections in infants: a spectrum of disease" *J. Pediatr. 76*, 405, 1970.

Torstenson, O. L., Meyer, W. J., Quie, P. G.: "Burn-wound infection with viruses" *New Eng. J. Med. 282*, 1272, 1970.

Tucker, E. S., Scofield, G. P.: "Hepato-adrenal necrosis: fatal systemic herpes simplex infection: review of literature and report of two cases" *Arch. Pathol 71*, 538, 1961.

Tuffli, G. A., Nahmias, A. J.: "Neonatal herpetic infection. Report of two premature infants treated with systemic use of idoxyridine" *Am. J. Dis. Child. 118*, 909, 1969.

Underwood, G. E.: "Activity of 1-beta-D-arabinofuranosylcytosine hydrochloride against herpes simplex keratitis" *Proc. Soc. Exp. Biol. Med. 11*, 661, 1962.

Underwood, G. E.: "Clinical evaluation of 4-2-nitro-1-(p-tolylthio) ethyl/ /acetonilide (U-3243) against cutaneous herpes simplex" *Ann. N.Y. Acad. Sci. 173*, 782, 1970.

Unna, P.: "On herpes progenitalis, especially in women" *J. Cut. Ven. Dis. 1*, 321, 1883.

Upton, A., Gumpert, J.: "Electroencephalography in diagnosis of herpes simplex encephalitis" *Lancet 1*, 650, 1970.

Upton, A., Barwick, D., Foster, B.: "Dexamethasone treatment in herpes simplex encephalitis" *Lancet 1*, 290, 1971.

Urbach, E.: "Herpes labialis. Erythema exudativum multiforme" *Zbl. f. Haut. u. Gesch Lechtrank. 46*, 413, 1933.

Urbach, E.: "Gesetzmessiger Zusammenhang zwischen Herpes labialis und Erythema exudativum multiforme" *Zbl. f. Haut. u. Geschlechtkrank 57*, 2, 1937.

Ustvedt, H. J.: "Erythema exudativum multiforme. The clinical picture" *Acta Med. Scand. 131*, 32, 1948.

Verini, M., Floretti, A., Casazza, A. M.: "Attivita in vitro di alcuni derivati distamicina A su virus erpetici" *Giorn. Mal. Inf. Paras. 24*, 11, 1972.

Vestergaard, B. F., Hornsleth, A., Pederson, S. N.: "Occurrence of herpes and adenovirus antibodies in patients with carcinoma of the cervix uteri" *Cancer 30*, 68, 1972.

Vivell, O., Hitzig, W. H., Cremer, H. J.: "Zu Klinik, Diagnose und Epidemiologie der Herpes-simplex Infectionen" *Helv. Paediatr. Acta. 12*, 2, 127, 1957.

Vortel, V., Herout, V.: "Generalieserte Infection mit dem virus des Herpes simplex bei Kindern" *Zbl. Allerg. Pathol. Anat. 96*, 51, 1957.

Vukas, A., Kon, V.: "Liječenje herpes simplex vakcinom influence" (Treatment of herpes simplex with influenza vaccine) *Medicina 3*, 25, 1966.

Wallis, C., Melnick, J. L.: "Photodynamic inactivation of animal viruses. A review" *Photochem. Photobiol. 4*, 159, 1965.

Ward, J. R., Clark, L.: "Primary herpes simplex virus infection of the fingers" *JAMA 176*, 3, 226, 1961.

Warren, W. S., Salvatore, M. A.: "Herpesvirus hominis infection at smallpox vaccination site" *JAMA 205*, 13, 931, 1968.

Wassermannova, V., Kubelka, V.: "Antiherpetička vakcina u oftalmologiji" (Antiherpetic vaccine in ophthalmology) *Čas. Oftalmologije 15*, 1, 1959.

Watson, D. H.: "Replication of the viruses: morphological aspects," pp. 133—159 in Kaplan, A. S. ed., *The Herpesviruses* (Academic Press, New York, 1973).

Weiss, J. F., Kibrick, S., Lever, W. F.: "Eczema herpeticum as complication of Darier's disease" *Ann. Int. Med. 62*, 1293, 1965.

Wenner, H. A.: "Complications of infantile eczema caused by the virus of herpes simplex" *Am. J. Dis. Child. 67*, 247, 1944.

Wentworth, B. B., Alexander, E. R.: "Seroepidemiology of infections due to members of the herpes group" *Am. J. Epid. 94*, 5, 496, 1971.

Wheeler, C. E.: "Further studies on the effect of neutralizing antibody upon the course of herpes simplex infections in tissue culture" *J. Immunol. 84*, 394, 1960.

Wheeler, C. E., Cabaniss, W.: "Epidemic cutaneous herpes simplex in wrestlers, herpes gladiatorum" *JAMA 194*, 9, 993, 1965.

Wheeler, C. E., Huffiness, W. D.: "Primary disseminated herpes simplex of the newborn" *JAMA 191*, 455, 1965.

Wheeler, C. E., Abelo, D. Č., Hill, C.: "Eczema herpeticum, primary and recurrent" *Arch. Dermatol. 93*, 162, 1966.

White, D. O., Shew, M. A., Howsman, K. G., Robertsen, I. F.: "Herpes virus infection of the cornea" *Med. J. Austral.* 2, 59, 1968.

Wilbanks, G. D., Campbell, J. A., Kaufmann, L. A.: "Cellular changes of normal human cervical epithelium infected in vitro with herpesvirus hominis type two (herpes simplex)" *Acta Cytol.* 14, 8, 538, 1970.

Wilcox, R. R.: "Necrotic cervicitis due to primary infections with the virus of herpes simplex" *Brit. Med. J.* 1, 610, 1968.

Wildy, P.: "Herpes: history and classification", pp. 1—22 in Kaplan, A. S., ed., *The Herpesviruses* (Academic Press, New York, 1973).

Wildy, P., Russell, W. C., Home, R. W.: "The morphology of herpesvirus" *Virology 12*, 204, 1960.

Williams, A., Jack, I.: "Hepatic necrosis in neonatal herpes simplex infection" *Med. J. Austral.*, 1, 392, 1955.

Wilt, J. C., Hendey, M. B., Stackew, W.: "Herpes simplex encephalitis" *Canad. Med. Assoc. 101*, 411, 1969.

Wilton, J. M. A., Ivanyi, L., Lehner, T.: "Cell-mediated immunity in herpes virus hominis infections" *Brit. Med. J. 18*, 723, 1972.

Witmer, R., Inomato, T.: "Electron microscopic observation of the iris in herpes uveitis" *Arch. Ophthalmol. 79*, 331, 1968.

Witzleben, C. L., Driscoll, S. G.: "Possible transplacental transmission of herpes simplex infections" *Pediatrics 36*, 192, 1965.

Wolinska, W., Melamed, M. R.: "Herpes genitalis in women attending Planned Parenthood in New York city" — *Acta Cytol. 14/5*, 239, 1970.

Womack, C. R., Randall, C. C.: "Erythema exudativum multiforme. Its association with viral infections" *Am. J. Med. 15*, 633, 1953.

Woolfe, A. B., Hoult, J. G.; in L. van Bogaert *et al.*, eds., *Encephalitides. Proceedings of a Symposium on the Neuropathology, Electroencephalography and Biochemistry of Encephalitides, Antwerp, 1959* (Amsterdam: Elsevier, 1961) pp. 315—324.

Wright, H. T., Miller, A.: "Fatal infection in a newborn infant due to the herpes simplex virus: report of a case diagnosed before death" *J. Pediatr. 67*, 130, 1965.

Wukelich, S. P.: "Primary herpes simplex infection of the finger: report of case" *J. Canad. Dent. Assoc. 38*, 3ᶜ, 1972.

Wyburn-Mason, R.: "Malignant change following herpes simplex" *Brit. Med. J. 2*, 615, 1957.

Yamamoto, T., Otani, S., Shiraku, H.: "A study of the evolution of viral infection in experimental herpes simplex encephalitis and rabies by means of fluorescent antibody" *Acta Neuropathol. 5*, 288, 1965.

Yang, J. P. S., Wentworth, B. B.: "Study of immune cytotoxicity with herpes virus hominis infected cells" *Proc. Soc. Exp. Biol. Med. 141*, 759, 1972.

Yang, J. P. S., Gale, J. L., Lee, G. C. Y.: "The cytotoxic effect of human immune sera on herpes virus hominis infected cells" *Proc. Soc. Exp. Biol. Med. 143*, 28, 1973.

Yen, S. S. C., Reagan, J. W., Rosenthal, M. S.: "Herpes simplex infection in the female genital tract" *Obstet. Gynecol. 25*, 479, 1965.

Yoshino, K., Taniguchi, S.: "Evaluation of the demonstration of complement requiring neutralising antibody as a means for early diagnosis of herpes virus infections" *J. Immunol. 96*, 196, 1966.

172

Zavoral, J. H., Ray, W. R., Kinnard, P. G., Nahmias, A. J.: "Neonatal herpetic infection. A fatal consequence of penile herpes in a serviceman" *JAMA* *213*, 1492, 1970.

Zisman, B., Hirsch, M. S., Allison, A. C.: "Selective effects of antimacrophage serum, silica and antilymphocyte of young adult mice" *J. Immunol. 104*, 1155, 1970.

Zuelzer, W. W., Stulberg, C. S.: "Herpes simplex virus as the cause of fulminating visceral disease and hepatitis in infancy. Report of eight cases and isolation of the virus in one case" *Am. J. Dis. Child. 83*, 421, 1952.

SUBJECT INDEX

AUTHOR INDEX

182

184

188

ADDENDUM

Since the completion of this book several new developments, especially in therapy, have made it necessary to modify the discussion above.

The most controversial method of inactivating herpes virus is the technique of *photodynamic inactivation*. The topical use of neutral red, followed by exposure to light, resulted in faster healing of herpetic lesions and reduction in the frequency of recurrences (Jarrat and Knox, 1975). Photo-inactivation therapy was also successful in the treatment of eczema herpeticum (Chang and Weinstein, 1975).

The first controlled studies showed that relapses were not prevented or appreciably reduced (Chang *et al.*, 1975). Li *et al.* (1975) pointed out that virus which has been inactivated photodynamically can transform cells to oncogenity in newborn hamsters. A causal relation between the technique of photo-inactivation and tumor induction is not proved in humans, however (R. H. Kaufman *et al.* 1977, 1978). The study of Friedrich *et al.* (1976), on the contrary, demonstrates that photodynamic dye light-therapy has not resulted in the development of epithelial atypia in a series of cases followed by vulval biopsy up to five years after treatment.

Photodynamic inactivation is no longer used in humans, because HSV may cause malignancies in man through a similar mechanism (Berger and Papa, 1977; Kopf *et al.*, 1978) and because recent reports of more extensive trials have shown that the treatment is not beneficial (Taylor and Doherty, 1975; Roome *et al.*, 1975; Myers *et al.*, 1976; Bartolomew *et al.*, 1977; R. H. Kaufman *et al.*, 1978).

Topical ether, though painful, did not shorten the duration of either primary or recurrent genital herpes and did not prevent or delay recurrent episodes (Corey *et al.*, 1978).

The topical use of *chloroform* does not appear sufficiently efficacious to recommend its routine use (Taylor *et al.*, 1977).

A nonionic surfactant active in vitro against HSV *nonoxynol-9* has been used for many years as a vaginal contraceptive. Recently considerable success has been described when the surfactant has been used for recurrent genital and labial herpes (Donsky, 1979); but another study of genital herpes, nonoxynol cream had no beneficial effect (Vontver *et al.*, 1979). Properly controlled double-blind trials have so far not been conducted.

Treatment of cutaneous HSV-type 2 infection with *8-methoxypsoralen* and *long wave ultraviolet light* in an animal model has demonstrated promising results (Oill et al., 1978).

A recently published method of treatment of genital herpes in the male with *ultrasound* and *zinc ointement* with *urea* and *tannic acid* requires further investigations and controlled studies (Fahim *et al.*, 1978).

Povidone-jodine (polyvinylpyrrolidone analog), the antiseptic paint, was used topically with some effect on herpetic lesions in noncontrolled studies (Friedrich and Masukawa, 1975; Woobridge, 1977).

Bonaphtone (6-naphtoquinone-1, 2) is reported in Russian medical literature to be therapeutically effective in experimental herpetic keratitis (Bogdanova *et al.*, 1975; Nikolaeva *et al.*, 1976).

The first reports mentioned in this book on the effectiveness of *phosphonoacetic acid* on experimental herpetic infection were confirmed in the more recently published articles. *Phosphonoacetic acid* was superior to IDU in experimental keratitis (Gordon *et al.*, 1977); more efficient than IDU, ara-A, ara-C, and ribavirin in experimental cutaneous herpes (Alenius and Oberg, 1978) and more successful than ara-A and arabinoside monophosphate in experimental genital herpes (Kern *et al.*, 1977). Phosphonoacetic acid or disodium phosphoacetate applied in experimental herpes encephalitis in rats resulted in much better reduction of titer of the virus in the brain and an increased rate of survival (Fitzwiliam and Griffith, 1976; Aoki *et al.*, 1979). There are no publications on the application of phosphonoacetic derivate in systemic human herpes virus infection.

Few interesting reports have been published on the relation between *nutrition* and *herpesvirus infection*. The use of water-soluble *bioflavonoid ascorbic acid* complex in the long-term treatment of recurrent herpes labialis in noncontrolled trials had moderate success in the mitigation of clinical manifestations and in reduction of the rate of recurrences (Terezhalmy *et al.*, 1978; Griffith *et al.*, 1978). The daily application of *aminoacid lysine*, in contrast to *arginine*, seems to supress the replication of virus but in reported clinical experiments may or may not prevent herpes recurrences (Kagan, 1974; Griffith *et al.*, 1978; Milman *et al.*, 1978).

The goal of *active immunization* against herpes virus infection is to prevent the primary exposure in children less than two years old with inactivated preparations of *HSV type 1*. This vaccine could not protect against *HSV type 2* infection because of the lack of cross-immunity. Consequently there is a need for later immunization of adolescents against HSV-2 infection (Smith, 1978). The problem in evaluating vaccines against herpes viruses is the same as in the drug therapy: to translate experience from an animal model to man is difficult because the pathogenesis can be very different in heterologous species (Horstmann, 1978).

The use of *inactivated HSV vaccines* against recurrent herpes virus infections is problematic, because individuals have both humoral and cellular immunity to HSV. The animal studies suggest that use of an inactivated HSV vaccine against recurrent infection is not efficacious (Scriba, 1978). However, some Russian experiences with the application of inactivated vaccine to prevent recurrences were to some degree promising in open trial (Shubladze *et al.*, 1978). Recently, heat-killed DNA containing vaccines — such as *Lupidon H* against HSV-1 and *Lupidon G* against HSV-2 — has been used in Germany. Encouraging results have been demonstrated in the treatment of secondary clinical exacerbations and in reduction of the rate of recurrences (Schmersahl and Rüdiger, 1975; Weitgasser, 1977). All these reported vaccines must be tested rigorously in well controlled studies before general use can be recommended.

A new approach to the study of vaccination is afforded by *subunit vaccines*, which are composed mainly of glycoproteins from the outer envelope of the virus. Such vaccines are free of nucleic acid, to avoid vaccine-induced malignancy. The vaccines might be successful against diseases caused by herpes viruses, but the use of subunit antigen against HSV is not yet licensed.

Another immunologic approach to prevention and therapy of herpetic infection is based on the enhancement of immune defense with specific or nonspecific stimulants. Trials are currently under way with BCG (Kern and Schiff, 1977; Fanta et al., 1977), with *transfer factor* (Rocha, 1977) and with *tilorene dihydrochloride*, an interferon inducer, in an experimental model (To-kumaru, 1975). A great number of articles have been recently published on the immunopotentiating activity of *levamisole*, an anthelminthic drug. The correlation between clinical and virus-specific immune responses following levamisole application, and its efficiency in an animal model, has been confirmed (O'Reilly et al., 1977; Friedlander et al., 1978). However, in experimental herpes encephalitis, levamisole in combination with ara-A had no effect on the course of the disease (Fischer et al., 1976). Despite some good results in open trials in humans (Adno, 1978; Haneke, 1979) and in controlled trials, levamisole was not useful in the treatment of recurrent herpes labialis (Russell et al., 1978). In other carefully controlled double-blind studies, on the contrary, levamisole proved to be effective (Kaufman and Vernell, 1977; Luderschmidt and Wolf, 1979). Further studies will be necessary to determine the value of immunopotentiation therapy of herpetic recurrences and particularly in the treatment of life-threatening herpes simplex infections. Because of the known tendency of levamisole to produce agranulocitosis, it is recommended that precaution be taken in the general use of levamisole in humans.

In experimental animals and in humans it has been confirmed that *interferon* and *interferon inducers* may be useful in treating herpetic infection, but this therapy is limited by many factors (insufficient concentration of applied interferon, the failure to alter the course of infection once the virus is established in target organs, etc.). The idea of using interferon to control herpetic infection in humans has been considered for many years but has not often been tested partly because of the advantage of new antiviral drugs over interferon and partly because suitable preparations of interferon were not available in past years. There now exist relatively potent preparations of interferon from primary human leukocytes (McGill et al., 1976). The application of homologous interferon in open and controlled studies in treatment of herpetic keratitis in humans is not encouraging when compared with other kinds of therapy, especially with respect to healing of ulcers (Jones et al., 1976; Sundmacher et al., 1976a; Sundmacher et al., 1976b). The results of the application of interferon for prevention of the recrudescence of herpetic lesions are also equivocal (Kaufman et al., 1976; Jones et al., 1976). Interferon works basically as a prophylactic agent and needs the support of further antiviral measures to be clinically effective (Guerra et al., 1977; Kern and Glasgow, 1977; Sundmacher et al., 1978). Combined administration of antiviral agents and humoral antibodies to HSV has resulted in enhanced protection in the animal model but warrants further investigation before its use in the therapy of human viral infections (Cho and Feng, 1977). In one study it was found that *ara-A* inhibits the beneficial effect of levamisole in experimental herpes encephalitis (Fischer et al., 1976). The topical action of combined therapy of human interferon and secretory immuno-globulin IgA was studied in a noncontrolled trial on herpetic keratitis patients, with promising results (Pena et al., 1978). Very interesting but questionable is the first report of intrathecal administration of interferon inducer *poly Ic (polyriboinosinic acid-polyribocytidilic acid)* in the case of neonatal generalized herpes virus infection with severe ocular involvement (Romano et al., 1978.)

Drugs currently or recently used in investigation for treatment of herpetic infection are mostly pyrimidine or purine derivatives. Unfortunately, therapy with these agents interferes with DNA metabolism of normal cells in a nonspecific way; therefore, treatment in man should be initiated with extreme caution because of possibly severe side effects (Alford and Whitley, 1976).

The most successful chemotherapeutic results have been with local treatment of HSV infections of the eye. All currently available antiviral substances for therapy of herpetic keratitis *(iodoxuridine, vidarabine, etc.)* are of greatest value in superficial forms but have little effect upon deep-seated stromal or uveal involvement. They offer treatment in acute exacerbations and cannot prevent recurrences.

The effectiveness of *iodoxuridine* as topical treatment for dendritic ulcers of the cornea caused by HSV is established beyond doubt. During therapy with IDU unresponsive cases and resistant isolates of herpes virus can be recovered (Jackson, 1978).

In double-blind studies there was no significant difference in healing time between iodoxuridine treated eyes and *adenin-arabinoside* treated eyes, but the marked adverse reactions to IDU were twofold more frequent (Pavan--Langston, 1975; Pavan-Langston and Buchanan, 1976; Markham *et al.*, 1977; Chin, 1978). It seems THAT ara-A is a safe and effective drug for treating herpetic keratitis, especially in iodoxuridine unresponsive and intolerant cases (Hindiuk *et al.*, 1975; McGill *et al.*, 1975; Abel *et al.*, 1975; O'Day *et al.*, 1976). Despite encouraging reports, the effectiveness of ara-A in herpetic iritis and deep stromal disease is problematic (Kaufman, 1975; McGill *et al.*, 1975). Treatment should often consist of the combined use of antiviral substances and debridement (cryotherapeutic) techniques, or corticosteroids (Colin, 1978; Tarakji *et al.*, 1978).

In marked contrast to the successful use of topical drug therapy for herpetic eye infection, local treatment of *mucocutaneous disease due to HSV-1 or 2* has resulted in no convincing evidence of its efficacy either for the therapy of individual attacks or for reduction of the frequency of recurrences. Topical use of adenine arabinoside against recurrent herpes labialis has a minimal effect on its clinical course, with no reduction of the frequency of episodes or the duration of lesions (Rowe *et al.*, 1979). The natural clinical course of either primary or recurrent genital herpetic infection in man and women was not influenced by local therapy with 3 percent ara-A in double-blind trials (Goodman *et al.*, 1975; Adams *et al.*, 1976; Hilton *et al.*, 1978). The need for effective and safe forms of local therapy for primary and recurrent mucocutaneous infections with HSV, especially when they are localized on the genitals, is necessarily acute.

Disseminated herpes in neonate or in *immuno-suppressed patients* and *herpetic encephalitis* require the use of systemic and urgent therapy. Initial clinical enthusiasm over *iodoxuridine* was so great that postponing therapy in order to conduct a controlled trial was excluded. The story of IDU as a systemic antiviral agent is therefore instructive as an example of an ethical dilemma that created an obstruction to the scientific approach. Additional investigations have shown, in fact, that IDU does not reach therapeutic concentrations in the human brain Lauter *et al.*, 1975). The occurrence of unacceptable myelosuppression and the failure of IDU therapy to prevent death led to the premature termination of two double blind studies in a Boston interhospital virus study (1975). The general view now seems to be that iodoxuridine is no longer indicated in the treatment of herpes encephalitis (Nüssli *et al.*, 1976; Bauer, 1977; Jackson, 1978).

The application of *cytosine-arabinoside* in herpes simplex encephalitis in children has met with partial success, but ara-C requires intolerable doses for the treatment of generalized and CNS infections in humans, and its use is not recommended (Brown and Bower, 1975; Lagerkvist and Ekelund, 1975).

Adenine-arabinoside, a purine derivate, possesses all the desirable characteristics of an antiviral agent: no incorporation in the host DNA; broad-spectrum activity against the DNA family of viruses; no resistance in vitro, rapid excretion, no immunosupression, low toxicity in significantly effective doses; and relatively low cost. Comparative treatment with cytosine-adenine in experimental herpes simplex virus encephalitis resulted in the long-term survival of a majority of infected animals in a series with ara-A (Griffith *et al.*, 1975). The results of a collaborative study of adenin-arabinoside in the United States suggest that in HSV encephalitis proved by brain biopsy, intravenous administration of ara-A at a dosage of 15 mg/kg body weight per day for 10 days reduced the mortality rate from 70 percent to 28 percent, although a high proportion of the survivors had neurological sequelae. The drug must be given early in the course of disease before the advent of coma (Whitley *et al.*, 1977; Taber *et al.*, 1977). Whitley *et al.* (1975) suggest that adenine arabinoside, eithin its nontoxic dose range, may be efficacious in the treatment of disseminated neonatal herpes virus infection provided the drug is given early in the course of the disease. Toxic effects from ara-A were nausea and vomiting, weight loss, weakness, megaloblastosis in bone marrow, tremors 5 to 7 days after the start of therapy, and thrombophlebitis at the intravenous site (Ross *et al.*, 1976). Adverse side reactions to ara-A were reversible and associated with a higher dose of the drug. Although adenin-arabinoside is in several ways superior to IDU, it has the disadvantage of rapid inactivation and poor solubility (Markham *et al.*, 1977; Theodoridis *et al.*, 1978). Adenine arabinoside has been released officially in the United States for use in the treatment of herpes simplex encephalitis.

General supportive treatment and nursing care must be of the highest quality, because patients with herpes encephalitis or disseminated herpes are greatly at risk from respiratory and cardiovascular complications (Longson and Bailey, 1977). In herpes encephalitis there is very often fatal cerebral oedema, which must be controlled. Specific virus chemotherapy could be insufficient without aggressive cerebral decompression. This decompression can be achieved surgically or medically by using mannitol or dexamethasone. The place of steroids in the therapy of herpes encephalitis is still a matter of dispute. Most authors agree that dexamethasone should be administered in large doses in all cases of herpes encephalitis (Longson and Bailey, 1977).

The results of supportive and antiviral drug therapy in disseminated herpes are very encouraging but far from the desirable goal of few or no sequelae.

Develoment of new antiviral drugs has been encouraged by the above facts: *Trifluorothymidine* (Trifluridine, F3T), with the generic name 5-trifluoremethyl-2 deoxyuridine, is pyrimidine nucleoside as IDU. The biologic activity of trifluridine is antimetabolic in the pathway of DNA synthesis. Its antitumor effect and antiviral activity was observed in experimental conditions (Bauer, 1977). In an animal model it was efficacious against herpes virus and in the treatment of experimental keratitis (Pavan-Langston and Langston, 1975). In controlled trials in humans, trifluromidine has demonstrated the same results (or better) as has IDU or ara-A in herpetic keratitis (Coster *et al.* 1976; Pavan--Langston and Foster, 1977; Laibson *et al.*, 1977; Travers and Patterson, 1978). Trifluridine has also been effective in resistant human herpetic keratitis that is unresponsive to topical IDU or ara-A therapy (Hindiuk *et al.*, 1978). Comparative therapy of experimental herpes simplex keratouveitis with adenine arabinoside drops and trifluiridine and iodoxuridine drops showed that ara-A (vidarabine) drops are not so effective as iodoxuridine or trifluiridine drops. However, ara-A (vidarabine) ointment was very effective (Pavan-Langston *et al.*, 1979).

Ribavirin, the medication in use against influenza, has been evaluated in vitro and in vivo on herpes virus, with moderate success (Allen *et al.*, 1977).

Adenino arabinoside monophosphate (Ara-AMO), a derivative of adenine arabinoside, manifested antiviral activity equivalent to ara-A against herpes viruses type 1 and 2 in tissue culture. Adenine arabinoside monophosphate in 20 percent solution was superior to a 3 percent solution of ara-A in experimental herpetic keratitis (Trobe *et al.*, 1976). Adenine ara-binoside monophosphate, because of its high solubility, permitted more concentrated solutions to be presented topically, and with adequate absorption by parenteral routes with smaller fluid loads than required for ara-A (Pavan-Langston *et al.*, 1976; Werner *et al.*, 1978). Trifluridine and adenin ara-binoside monophosphate were compared in animal models of herpes simplex stromal keratitis (McNeill and Kaufman, 1979). When given early and frequently, these drugs suppressed the disease, but later in the clinical course neither drug had an appreciable effect. Despite its proven activity against HSV in vitro and in vivo on the animal model, topical use of adenine arabinoside monophosphate in controlled study of the treatment of recurrent herpes labialis in humans was ineffective. This may be due to failure of the drug to penetrate the skin (Spruance *et al.*, 1979).

9-beta-D-arabinofuranosyladenine-5-phosphate (Ara-A5-P) is a very soluble derivate of adenin arabinoside. It is well tolerated; it has proven antiherpetic activity in vitro, and it has been used successfully in the topical treatment of herpes-simplex-induced keratitis in rabbits (Falcon and Jones, 1977). The preliminary results of therapy with this drug in experimental herpes encephalitis in mice were also promising (Adams and Cameron, 1977).

Acycloguanosine, acyclic antimetabolite — an analog of gyanosine (9-2-hydroxyethoxymethyl) guanine, was found to be the most active agent against herpes growth in cell culture (100 times as active as ara-A) and to have marked antiviral activity in animal models of herpes simplex virus infection associated with very low toxicity (Annexton, 1978; Schaeffer *et al.*, 1978; Kaufman *et al.*, 1978). The comparison with IDU and ara-A in experimental animal keratitis has demonstrated the significantly better advantage of acycloguanosine (Pavan-Langston *et al.*, 1979). Recently, in an open clinical study, the efficacy of acycloguanosine in human herpetic keratitis was demonstrated (Jones *et al.*, 1979).

Systemic antiviral chemotherapy is still in its infancy. Every research has three principal phases. In the first preclinical phase the extrapolation of results from the animal model to man is diffficult, either because of the species difference in metabolism of drugs or because the host-parasite relationship is different. For instance, experimental encephalitis is always a primary infection, but in man, herpes encephalitis is a reactive phenomenon (Longson and Bailey, 1977). Uncontrolled use of an experimental compound destined for systemic use is the second phase of investigation. Anecdotal or serial observations carry the risk of wrong results, the most common ones of which are unsatisfied diagnostic procedures (for instance, the biopsy did not prove encephalitis) or the existence of many different criteria for evaluating the applied therapy. Spruance *et al.* (1977) performed quantitative and objective measurements in the clinical course of recurrent herpes which could be used in monitoring the efficacy of antiviral chemotherapy. Phase 3 double-blind and randomized trials were often disparate from the results of noncontrolled studies (Goodheart and Guinan, 1979). "The pioneering mistakes in the past, through emphasizing need, may have provided the impetus for more fruitful accomplishments to come" (Alford and Whitley, 1976).

BIBLIOGRAPHY TO ADDENDUM

Abel, R., Kaufman, H. E., Sugar, J.: "Intravenous adenine arabinoside a-gainst herpes simplex" *Am. J. Ophthalmolog. 79*, 659, 1975.

Adams, D. H., Cameron, K. R.: "Derivative of adenine arabinoside in experimental herpes encephalitis" *Lancet*, 760, 1977.

Adams, H. G., Benson, E. A., Alexander, E. R., Vontver, A., Remington, M. A., Holmes, K. K.: "Genital herpetic infection in men and women: clinical course and effect of topical application of adenine arabinoside" *J. Infect. Dis. 133*, Suppl. A, 151, 1976.

Adno, J.: "Levamisole and treatment of herpesvirus hominis infections: a case report" *S. Afr. Med. J., 53*, 547, 1978.

Alenius, S., Oberg, B.: "Comparison of the therapeutic affects of live antiviral agents on cutaneous herpesvirus infection in guinea pigs" *Arch. Virol. 58*, 227, 1978.

Alford, C. A., Whitley, R. J.: "Treatment of infection due to herpesvirus in humans: a critical review of the state of the art" *J. Infect. Dis. 133*, Suppl. A, 101, 1976.

Allen, L. B., Wolf, S. M., Hintz, C. J., Huffman, J. H., Sidwell, R. W.: "Effect of ribavirin on type 2 herpesvirus hominis (HVH/2) in vitro and in vivo" *Ann. NY Acad. Sci. 284*, 247, 1977.

Annexton, M.: "Promising new antiherpes agent being tested in humans" *JAMA, 240*, 2231, 1978.

Aoki, F. Y., Trèpanier, G., Lussier, G.: "Intracerebroventricular and intraperitoneal disodium phosphoacetate treatment of herpes simplex virus type 1 experimental encephalitis" *J. Infect. Dis. 130*, 158, 1979.

Bartolomew, R. S., Clarke, M., Phillips, C. I.: "Dye light" induced photo sensitization of herpes virus: clinical trial on humans" *Trans. Ophthalmol. Soc. UK. 97*, 508, 1977.

Bauer, D. J.: "The specific treatment of virus diseases" MTP, Lancaster, 1977.

Berger, R. S., Papa, C. M.: "Photodye herpes therapy Casandra confirmed?" *JAMA 238*, 133, 1977.

Bogdanova, N. S., Nikolaeva, I. S., Pershin, G. N.: "Chemotherapeutic activity of bonafton in exeprimental herpetic keratitis in rabbits" *Farmakol. Toksikol. 38*, 728, 1975. (RUS)

Brown, R. S., Bower, B. D.: "Neonatal disseminated herpes simplex virus infection with encephalitis treated with cytosine arabinoside" *Dev. Med. Child. Neurol. 17*, 493, 1975.

Chang, T. W., Weinstein, L.: "Eczema herpeticum: Treatement with methylene blue and light" *Arch. Dermatol. 111*, 1174, 1975.

Chang, T. W., Fiumara, N., Weinstein, L.: "Genital herpes treatement with methylene blue and light exposure" *Int. J. Dermatol. 14*, 1, 69, 1975.

Chin, G. N.: "Treatement of herpes simplex keratitis with idoxuridine and vidarabine: a double blind study" *Ann. Ophthalmol. 10*, 1171, 1978.

Cho, C. T., Feng, K. K.: "Synergistic effects of antiviral agents and humoral antibodies in experimental herpesvirus hominis encephalitis" *Ann. NY Acad. Sci. 284*, 321, 1977.

Colin, J.: "Ocular herpes: Therapeutic aspect" *Nouv. Presse Med. 7*, 2949, 1978. (FR.)

Corey, L., Reeves, W., Chiang, W. T., Vontver, L. A., Remington, M., Winter, C., Holmes, K. K.: "Ineffectiveness of topical ether for the treatment of genital herpes simplex virus infection" *N. Engl. J. Med. 299*, 237, 1978.

Coster, D. J., McKinnon, J. R., McGill, J. I., Jones, B. R., Fraunfelder, F. T.: "Clinical evaluation of edenine arabinoside and trifluorthymidine in the treatment of corneal ulcer caused by herpes simplex virus" *J. Infect. Dis. 133*, Suppl. A, 173, 1976.

De la, Pena, N. C., Diaz, A., Damel, A., Bal, E., Puricelli, L., Ejden, J., De Lustig, E. S.: "Combined therapy of human interferon (HI) and secretory immunoglobulin (S-IgA) in the treatment of human herpetic keratitis" *Biomedicine 28*, 104, 1978.

Donsky, H. J.: "Nonoxynol 9 cream for genital herpes simplex" *N. Engl. J. Med. 300*, 371, 1979.

Donsky, H. J.: "Treatment of genital herpes" *N. Engl. J. Med. 300*, 338, 1979.

Fahim, M., Brawner, T., Millikan, L., Nickell, M., Hall, D.: "New treatment for herpes simplex virus type 2 (ultrasound and zinc, urea, tannic acid ointement), Part I, Male patients" *J. Med. 9*, 245, 1978.

Falcon, M. G., Jones, B. R.: "Herpes simplex keratitis: animal model to guide the selection and optimal delivery of antiviral chemotherapy" *J. Antimicrob. Chemotherapy 3*, Suppl. A, 83, 1977.

Fanta, D., Dostal, V., Reiss-Gutfreund, R.: "BCG therapy of recurrent herpes simplex type 1 and 2 (HSV 1 and 2)" *Z. Hautkr. 52*, 1099,1977. (GER)

Fischer, G. W., Balk, M. W., Crumrie, M. H., Bass, J. W.: "Imunopotentiation and antiviral chemotherapy in a suckling rat model of herpes encephalitis" *J. Infect. Dis. 133*, Suppl. A 2, 171, 1976.

Fitzwiliam, J. F., Griffith, J. F.: "Experimental encephalitis caused by herpes simplex virus: comparison of treatment with tilorone hydrochloride and phosphonoacetic acid" *J. Infect. Dis. 133*, Suppl. A, 221, 1976.

Friedlander, M. H., Smolin, G., Okumoto, M.: "The treatment of herpetic reinfection with levamisole" *Am. J. Ophthalmol. 86*, 245, 1978.

Friedrich, E. G., Masukawa, T.: "Effect of povidone-iodine on herpes genitalis" *Obst. Gynecol. 45*, 337, 1975.

Friedrich, E. G., Kaufman, R. E., Lynch, P. J., Woodruff, D.: "Vulvar histology after neutral red photoinactivation of herpes simplex virus" *Obst. Gynecol. 48*, 564, 1976.

Goodheart, G. L., Guinan, M. E.: "Treatment of genital herpes simplex" *N. Engl. J. Med. 300*, 1338, 1979.

Goodman, E. L., Luby, J. P., Johnson, M. T.: "Prospective double-blind evaluation of topical adenine arabinoside in male herpes progenitalis" *Antimicrob. Agents. Chemother. 8*, 693, 1975.

198

Gordon, Y. J., Lahav, M., Photiou, S., Becker, Y.: "Effect of phosphonoacetic acid in the treatment of experimental herpes simplex keratitis" Br. J. Ophthalmol. *61*, 506, 1977.

Griffith, J. F., Fitzwilliam, J. F., Casagrande, S., Butler, R. S.: "Experimental herpes simplex virus encephalitis: comparative effects of treatment with cytosine arabinoside and adenine arabinoside" J. Infect. Dis. *132*, 506, 1975.

Griffith, R. S., Norins, A. L., Kagan, C.: "A multicentered study of lysine therapy in herpes simplex infection" Dermatologica *156*, 257, 1978.

Guerra, R., Galin, M. A., Frezzotti, R.: "Use of interferon in eye infections of man" Tex. Rep. Biol. Med. *35*, 497, 1977.

Haneke, E.: "Levamisole therapy under different dermatological indications" Z. Hautkr. *54*, 408, 1979. (GER)

Hilton, A. L., Bushell, T. E., Waller, D., Bright, J.: "A trial of adenine arabinoside in genital herpes" Br. J. Vener. Dis. *54*, 50, 1978.

Hindiuk, R. A., Hull, D. S., Schultz, R. O., Chin, G. N.: "Adenine arabinoside in idoxuridine unresposive and intolerant herpetic keratitis" Am. J. Ophthalmol. 79, 655, 1975.

Hindiuk, R. A., Charlin, R. E., Alpren, T. V., Schultz, R. O.: "Trifluridine in resistant human herpetic keratitis" Arch. Ophtalmol. 96, 1839, 1978.

Horstmann, D. M.: "Immunization against viral infections" in Rothschild, H., Allison, F., Howe, C.: Human diseases caused by viruses — recent developments, Oxford Univer. press, New York, 1978.

Jackson, G. G.: "Chemotherapy" in Rothschild, H., Allison, F., Howe, C.: "Human diseases caused by viruses — recent developments" Oxford Univ. Press, New York, 1978.

Jarrat, M., Knox, J.: "The photodynamic effect in herpes simplex: a review" Hautarzt 26, 345, 1975. (GER.)

Jones, B. R., Coster, D. J., Falcon, M. G., Cantell, K.: "Clinical trial of topical interferon and ulcerative viral keratitis" J. Infect. Dis. *133*, Suppl. A, 169, 1976.

Jones, B. R., Coster, D. J., Fison, P. N., Thompson, G. M., Gobo, L. M., Falcon, M. G.: "Efficacy of acycloguanosine (Wellcome 248U) against herpes simplex corneal ulcers" Lancet *1*, 243, 1979.

Kagan, C.: "Lysine therapy of herpes simplex" Lancet *1*, 174, 1974.

Kaufman, H. E.: "Systemic therapy of ocular herpes" Int. Ophthalmol. clin. *15*, 163, 1975.

Kaufman, H. E., Varnell, E. D.: "Lack of levamysole effect on experimental herpes keratitis" Invest. Ophthalmol. Vis. Sci. *16*, 1148, 1977.

Kaufman, H. E., Meyer, R. F., Laibson, P. R.: "Human leukocyte interferon for the prevention of recurrences of herpetic keratitis" J. Infect. Dis. *133*, 165, 1976.

Kaufman, H. E., Varnell, E. D., Centifanto, Y. M., Rheinstrom, S. D.: "Effect of 9-(2-hydroxyethoxymethyl) guanine on herpes-virus-induced keratitis and iritis in rabbits" Antimicrob. Agents Chemother. 14, 842, 1978.

Kaufman, R. H., Bertner, E. W., Friedrich, E. G.: "Casandra still a myth" JAMA *238*, 2368, 1977.

Kaufman, R. H., Adam, E., Mirković, R. R., Melnick, J. L., Young, R. L.: "Treatment of genital herpes simplex virus infection with photodynamic inactivation" Am. J. Obstet. Gynecol. *132*, 861, 1978.

Kern, A. B., Schiff, B. L.: "Treatment of herpes simplex infections" *Arch. Dermatol. 113*, 1463, 1977.

Kern, E. R., Glasgow, L. A.: "Effect of interferon on systemic herpesvirus infections" *Tex. Rep. Biol. Med. 35*, 472, 1977.

Kern, E. R., Richards, J. T., Overall, J. C., Glasgow, L. A.: "Genital herpesvirus hominis infection in mice: II Treatment with phosphonoacetic acid, adenine arabinoside and adenine arabinoside 5-monophosphate" *J. Infect. Dis. 135*, 557, 1977.

Kopf, A. W., Ackerman, A. B., Wade, T., Bart, R. S.: "Photodye herpes therapy" *JAMA 239*, (7): 615, 1978.

Lagerkvist, B., Ekelund, H.: "Cytarabine treatement of herpes simplex encephalitis in infants and small children: a report on three cases with short review of the literature" *Scand. J. Infect. Dis. 7*, 81, 1975.

Laibson, P. R., Arentsen, J. J., Mazzanti, W. D., Eiferman, R. A.: "Double controlled comparison of IDU and trifluorothymidine in thirty-three patients with superficial herpetic keratitis" *Trans. Am. Ophthalmol. Soc. 75*, 316, 1977.

Lauter, C. B., Bailey, E. J., Lerner, A. M.: "Absence ofidoxuridine and persistence of herpes simplex virus in brains of patients being treated for encephalitis" *Proc. Soc. Exp. Biol. Med. 150*, 23, 1975.

Li, J. H., Jerkowsky, M., Rapp, F.: "Demonstration of oncogenic potential of mammalia cells transformed by DNA-containing viruses following photodynamic inactivation" *Int. J. Cancer 15*, 190, 1975.

Longson, M., Bailey, A. S.: "Herpes encephalitis" in Waterson, A. P. "Recent advances in clinical virology" Churchill Livingstone, Edinburgh, 1977.

Luderschmidt, C., Wolf, H. H.: "Management of recurrent herpes simplex using levamisole" *Hautarzt 30*, 21, 1979. (GER)

Markham, R. H., Carter, C., Scobie, M. A., Metcalf, C., Easty, D. L.: "Double blind clinical trial of adenine arabinoside and idoxuridine in herpetic corneal ulcers" *Trans. Ophthalmol. Soc. UK 97*, 333, 1977.

McGill, J. I., Coster, D., Frauenfelder, T., Holt-Wilson, A. D., Wiliams, H., Jones, B. R.: "Adenine arabinoside in the management of herpetic keratitis" *Trans. Ophthalmol. Soc. 95*, 246, 1975.

McGill, J. I., Collins, P., Cantel, K., Jones, B. R., Finter, N. B.: "Optimal schedules for use of interferon in the corneas of rabbits with herpes simplex keratitis" *J. Infect. Dis. 133*, Suppl. A, 13, 1976.

McNeill, J. I., Kaufman, H. E.: "Local antivirals in a herpes simplex stromal keratitis model" *Arch. Ophthalmol. 97*, 727, 1979.

Milman, N., Scheibel, J., Jessen, O.: "Failure of lysine treatment in recurrent herpes simplex labialis" *Lancet 2*, 942, 1978.

Myers, M. G., Oxman, M. N., Clark, J. E.: "Photodynamic inactivations in recurrent infections with herpes simplex virus" *J. Infect. Dis. 133*, 145, 1976.

Nikolaeva, I. S., Kutchak, S. N., Bogdanova, N. S., Pershin, G. N.: "Pathomorphological study of antiviral chemotherapeutic effectiveness of bonaphton under experimental conditions" *Farmakol. Toksikolog. 39*, 336, 1976.

Nüssli, R., Kind, H. P., Duc, G.: "Herpes simplex encephalitis in Neugeborenen: therapy mit 5-jodo-2-deoxyuridine" *Eur. J. Pediatr. 112*, 131, 1976.

O'Day, D. M., Poirier, R. H., Jones, D. B., Elliott, J. H.: "Vidarabine therapy of complicated herpes simplex keratitis" *Am. J. Ophthalmol. 81*, 642, 1976.

Oill, P. A., Galpin, J. E., Fox, M. A., Guze, L. B.: "Treatment of cutaneous herpesvirus hominis type 2 infection with 8-methoxypsoralen and long wave ultraviolet light in guinea pigs" *J. Infect. Dis. 137*, 715, 1978.

O'Reilly, R. J., Chibaro, A., Wilmot, R., Lopez, C.: "Correlation of clinical and virus-specific immune resposes following levamisole therapy of recurrent herpes progenitalis" *Ann. NY Acad. Sci. 284*, 161, 1977.

Pavan-Langston, D.: "Clinical evaluation of adenine arabinoside and idoxuridine in the treatment of ocular herpes simplex" *Am. J. Ophthalmol. 80*, 495, 1975.

Pavan-Langston, D., Langston, R. H.: "Recent advances in antiviral therapy" *Int. Ophthalmol. Clin. 15*, 89, 1975.

Pavan-Langston, D., North, R. D., Geary, P. A.: "Ara-AMP: a highly soluble new antiviral drug" *Ann. Ophthalmol. 8*, 571, 1976.

Pavan-Langston, D., Buchanan, R.: "Vidarabine therapy of simple one IDR--complicated herpetic keratitis" *Trans. Am. Acad. Ophthalmolog. Otolaryngol. 81*, 813, 1976.

Pavan-Langston, D., Foster, C. S.: "Trifluorthymidine and idoxuridine therapy of ocular herpes" *Am. J. Ophthalmol. 84*, 818, 1977.

Pavan-Langston, D., Lass, J., Campbell, R.: "Antiviral drops: comparative therapy of experimental herpes simplex keratitis" *Arch. Ophthalmol. 97*, 1132, 1979.

Rocha, H.: "Transfer factor in ophthalmology" *Klin. Monatsbl. Augenheilkd 171*, 63, 1977. (GER)

Romano, A., Kaplinsky, C., Frand, M., Rotem, Y., Stein, R.: "Systemic and topical use of poly IC in treatment of generalized neonatal herpes simplex infection with severe ocular involvement" *J. Pediatr. Ophthalmol. Strabismus 15*, 239, 1978.

Roome, A. P., Tinkler, A. E., Hilton, A. L., Montefiore, D. G., Waller, D.: "Neutral red with photoinactivation in the treatment of herpes genitalis" *Br. J. Vener. Dis. 51*, 130, 1975.

Ross, A. H., Julia, A., Balakrishnan, C.: "Toxicity of adenine arabinoside in humans" *J. Infect. Dis. 133*, Suppl. A, 192, 1976.

Rowe, N. H., Brooks, S. L., Young, S. K., Spencer, J., Petrick, T. J., Buchanan, R. A., Drach, J. C., Shipman, C.: "A clinical trial of topically applied 3 percent vidarabine against recurrent herpes labialis" *Oral. Surg. 47*, 142, 1979.

Russell, A. S., Brisson, E., Grace, M.: "A double-blind, controlled trial of levamisole in the treatment of recurrent herpes labialis" *J. Infect. Dis. 137*, 597, 1978.

Schaeffer, H. J., Beauchamp, L., De Miranda, P., Elion, G. B., Bauer, D. J., Collins, P.: "9-(2-hydroxyethoxymethyl) guanine activity against viruses of the herpes group" *Nature 272*, 583, 1978.

Schmersahl, P., Rüdiger, G.: "Results of treatment with the herpes simplex antigen Lupidon H resp. Lupidon G" *Z. Hautkra. 50*, 105, 1975 (GER.).

Scriba, M.: "Animal studies on the efficacy of an inactivated herpes simplex virus vaccine against recurrent herpes infection" *Infection 6*, 137, 1978.

Shubladze, A. K., Zaitseva, N. S., Maevskaia, T. M., Cheglakov, I. A., Muravèva, T. V.: "Mechanism of specific vaccino therapy in ocular herpes simplex" *Vopr. Virusol. 1,* 63, 1978. (RUS)

Smith, J. W.: „Herpesviruses" in Rothschild, H., Allison, F., Howe, C.: "Human diseases caused by viruses — recent developments" Oxford Univ. Press, New York, 1978.

Spruance, S, L., Overall, J. C., Kern, E. R., Krueger, G. G., Pliam, V., Miller, W.: "The natural history of recurrent herpes simplex labialis: implications for antiviral therapy" *N. Engl. J. Med. 297,* 69, 1977.

Spruance, S. L., Crumpacker, C. S., Hainess, H., Bader, C., Mehr, K., MacCalman, J., Schnipper, L. E., Klauber, M. R., Overall, J. C.: "Ineffectiveness of topical adenine arabinoside 5-monophosphate in the treatment of recurrent herpes simplex labialis" *N. Engl. J. Med. 300,* 1180, 1979.

Sundmacher, R., Neumann-Haefelin, D., Cantell, K.: "Successful treatment of dendritic keratitis with human leukocyte interferon: a controlled clinical study" *Albrecht von Graefes Arch. Klin. Ophthalmol. 201,* 39, 1976a.

Sundmacher, R., Neumann-Haefelin, D., Manthey, K. F., Müller, O.: "Interferon in treatment of dendritic keratitis in humans: A preliminary report" *J. Infect. Dis. 133,* Suppl. A, 160, 1976b.

Sundmacher, R., Cantell, K., Haug, P., Neumann-Haefelin, D.: "Role of debridement end interferon in the treatment of dendritic keratitis" *Albrecht Von Graefes Arch. Klin. Ophtalmol. 207,* 77, 1978.

Taber, L. H., Geenberg, S. B., Perez, F. I., Couch, R. B.: "Herpes simplex encephalitis treated with vidarabine (adenine arabinoside)" *Arch. Neurol. 34,* 608, 1977.

Tarakji, M. S., Matta, C. S., Shamas, H. F.: "Cryotherapy of herpes simplex keratitis" *Ann. Ophthalmolog. 10,* 1557, 1978.

Taylor, P. K., Doherty, N. R.: "Comparison of the treatment of herpes genitalis in men with proflavin photoinactivation, idoxuridine ointment and normal saline" *Br. J. Vener. Dis. 51,* 125, 1975.

Taylor, C. A., Hondley, J. O., Greer, K. E., Gwaltney, J. M.: "Topical treatment of herpes labialis with chloroform" *Arch. Dermatol. 113,* 1550, 1977.

Terezhalmy, G. T., Bottomley, W. K., Pelleu, G. B.: "The use of water soluble bioflavonoid-ascorbic acid complex in the treatment of recurrent herpes labialis" *Oral. Surg. 45,* 56, 1978.

Theodoridis, A., Sivenas, C., Vagena, A., Capetanakis, J.: "Double blind trial in the treatment of herpes simplex and herpes zoster with adenine arabinoside and idoxuridine" *Arch. Dermatol. Res. 262,* 173, 1978.

Tokumaru, T.: "The mode of inhibition of herpes simplex and vesicular stomatitis and ocular viral infections in the rabbit and hamster by an interferon inducer tiloron dihydrochloride" *Res. Commun. Chem. Pathol. Pharmacol. 11,* 289, 1975.

Travers, J. P., Patterson, A.: "A controlled trial of adenine arabinoside and trifluorothymidine in herpetic keratitis" *J Int. Med. Res. 6,* 102, 1978.

Trobe, J. D., Centifanto, Y., Zam, U. S., Varnell, E., Kaufman, H. E.: "Antiherpes activity of adenine arabinoside monophosphate" *Invest. Ophthalmol. 15,* 196, 1976.

Vontver, L. A., Reeves, W. C., Rattray, M., Corey, L., Remington, M. A., Tolentino, E., Schweid, A., Holmes, K. K.: "Clinical course and diagnosis of genital herpes simplex virus infection and evaluation of topical surfactant therapy" *Am. J. Obst. Gynecol. 1335,* 548, 1979.

202

Weitgasser, H.: "Controlled clinical study of the herpes antigens Lupidon H and Lupidon G" *Z. Hautkr.* *52*, 116, 25, 1977. (GER)

Werner, G. T., Bömer, H., Metzger, E., Sauer, O., Scheder, H., Schubert, E., Teuner, I.: "The virostatic effect of adenine arabinoside monophosphate experimental findings and preliminary clinical experiences" *Forschr. Med.* *96*, 1599, 1978. (GER)

Whitley, R. J., Chien, L. T., Alford, C. A.: "Neonatal herpes simplex virus infection" *Int. Ophtalmol. Clin.* *15*, 141, 1975.

Whitley, R. J., Soong, S. J., Dolin, R., Galasso, G. J., Chien, L. T.: "Adenine arabinoside therapy of biopsy proved herpes simplex encephalitis: national institute of allergy and infectious diseases collaborative antiviral study" *New. Engl. J. Med., 297*, 289, 1977.

Woobridge, P.: "The use of betadine antiseptic paint in the treatment of herpes simplex and herpes zoster" *J. Int. Med. Res. 5*, 378, 1977.